The Complete Book of Braids

Creative New Ways to Braid, Twist and Roll Your Hair

Linda Shields Ksiazek

Longmeadow Press

For Richard, Nicholas, and Whitney

Hair Design and Styles – Linda Shields Ksiazek
Photography – Anthony Badami
Publication Design & Graphics – M. Scott Mussett
Editors – Frank Christopher, Laird Bibler
Manuscripting – Becky Anderson

Special thanks to April Lauchner for her research on the Fishtail, and her styling assistance during the photo sessions. Also a special thanks to Scott Mussett for all his time and useful suggestions.

Cover design by David C. Merrell
Library of Congress Cataloging-in-Publication Data
ISBN: 0-681-41128-7
Printed in United States of America
First Edition
0   9   8   7   6   5   4

Introduction

This is a handbook for anyone who would like to learn new ways to style their hair. This book contains forty-five different braids, twists, rolls, and tucks to try on your hair with easy-to-follow, step-by-step instructions.

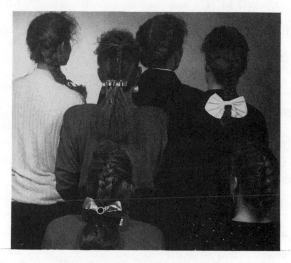

Acknowledgements

I would like to thank the models in the book. Their beautiful hair is an inspiration to all.

Models

Julie Ewing	April Lauchner
Cris Baugh	Denise Pratt
Lavon Melton	Linda Ksiazek
Danielle Richards	Caitilin Pratt
Whitney Ksiazek	Becky Anderson
Gina Price	Zena Pieters

Table of Contents

The Original Braid

The French Braid

The Twist

The Fishtail

The Roll

Braid Free

The Unbraid

The
Original

HE ORIGINAL THE ORIGINAL THE ORIGINAL THE ORIGINAL THE ORIGINAL THE ORIGINAL THE ORIGINAL THE ORIGINAL THE ORIGINAL

Introduction

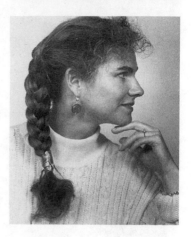

The Original Braid is a basic and simple braid to learn.

Even though this braid is the easiest one to do, there are many hairstyle variations which make this braiding technique invaluable.

The following chapter contains hairstyles using the Original Braid technique.

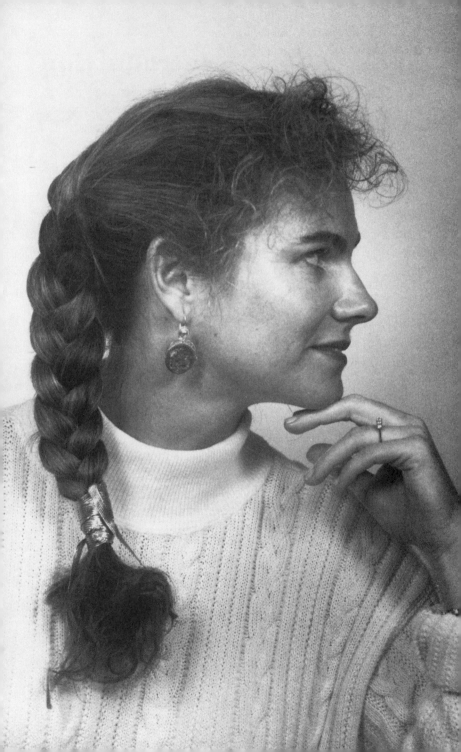

The Original

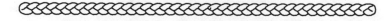

1 Divide your hair into three equal sections across the back of your head.

2 Place the right section over the middle section.

3 Place the left section over the new middle section.

4 Repeat steps 2 and 3 until you reach the desired length.

5 Secure with a covered band or hair clip. •

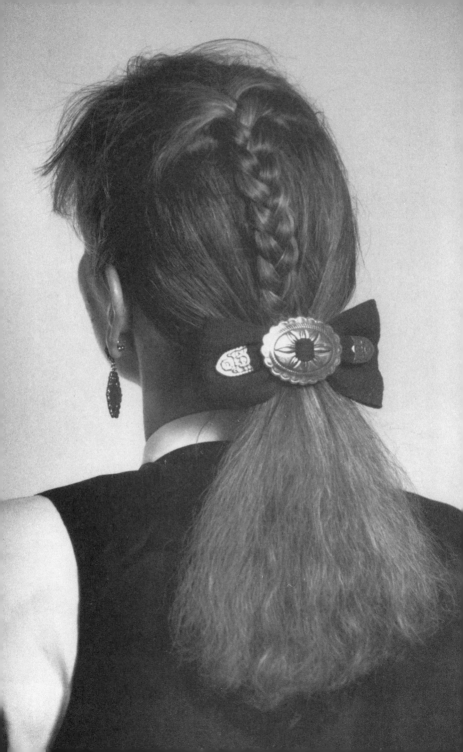

The Braid into a Ponytail

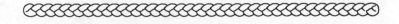

1 Gather the top one-third portion of your hair at the top of your head into one section. Leave the bottom two-thirds of your hair hanging free.

2 Divide this top section into three equal sections.

3 Braid this section, following the Original Braid method described on page 3. Braid until you reach the base of your hairline.

4 Gather and band the free hanging hair and braided section into a ponytail. Keep the small braided section in the center of your gathered ponytail.   •

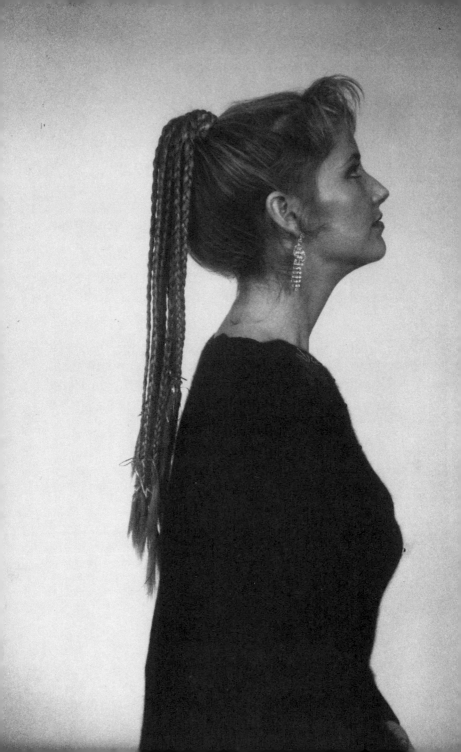

Lots of Braids

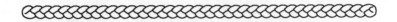

1 Gather and band all of your hair into a ponytail at the crown of your head.

2 Divide your hair into four to ten separate sections. The number of sections depends on the
thickness of your hair. The thicker your hair
the more braids you will want.

3 Braid each of the sections, following the Original Braid method described on page 3.

4 Secure the end of each braid with colored
bands, ribbons, or beads. Wrap one of the
braids around the top originating point to hide
the large band securing the ponytail.   •

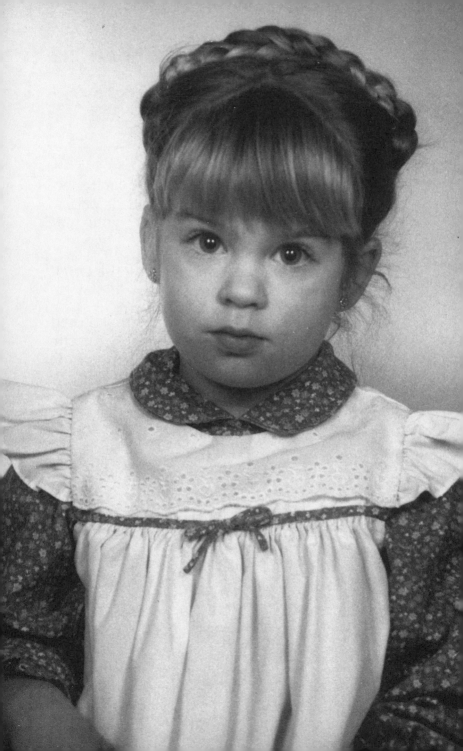

Little Dutch Girl

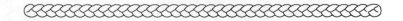

1   Part your hair into two sections from your fore-
    head to the base of your hairline. Loosely band
    one section while working on the other sec-
    tion.

2   Braid the free hanging section, using the Origi-
    nal Braid method described on page 3. Braid all
    the way to the ends and secure with a band.

3   Repeat step 2 with the second section.

4   Pull one finished braid upward over the top of
    your head, toward the opposite ear. Tuck the
    very end of the braid under itself and secure
    the braid with hairpins.

5   Repeat step 4 with the second braid. Lay the
    second braid alongside the first braid. Tuck the
    end under itself and secure with hairpins.   •

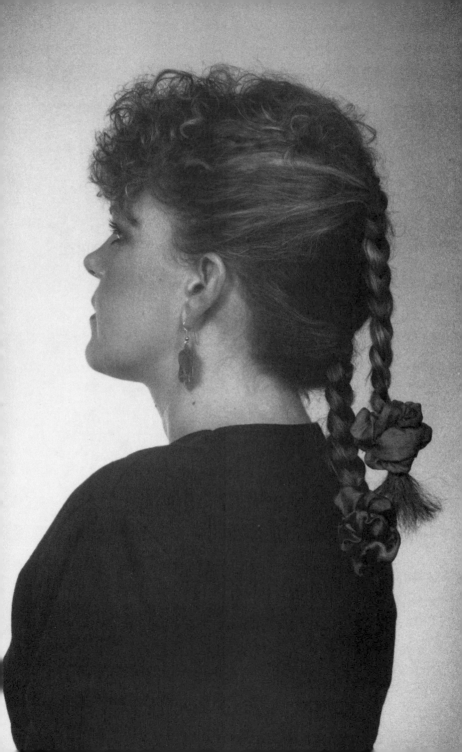

Original Piggyback

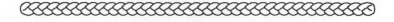

1 Divide your hair into two equal sections, with the part running horizontally from ear to ear. The top half of the hair, from ear to ear and above is section 1. The bottom half of the hair, from ear to ear and below is section 2.

2 Secure section 2 with a clip or band while working with section 1.

3 Braid section 1, using the Original Braid technique described on page 3. Braid entire length of hair. Secure with covered elastic band. Clip this braid out of the way while working on section 2.

4 Braid section 2 to its entire length and secure with a band.

5 Unclip section 1 and let it fall on top of the second braid.   •

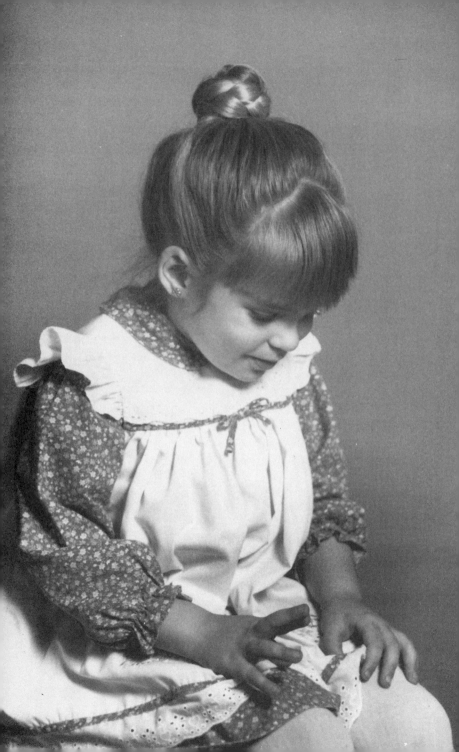

The Ballerina

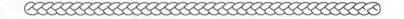

1 Gather all your hair into a high ponytail at the crown of your head.

2 Braid all of the hair, following the directions for the Original Braid method on page 3. Braid the entire length of hair. Secure end of braid with a covered elastic band.

3 Wrap the single braid around the top of your head in a circular motion. Tuck the end of the braid under itself, and secure with hairpins. •

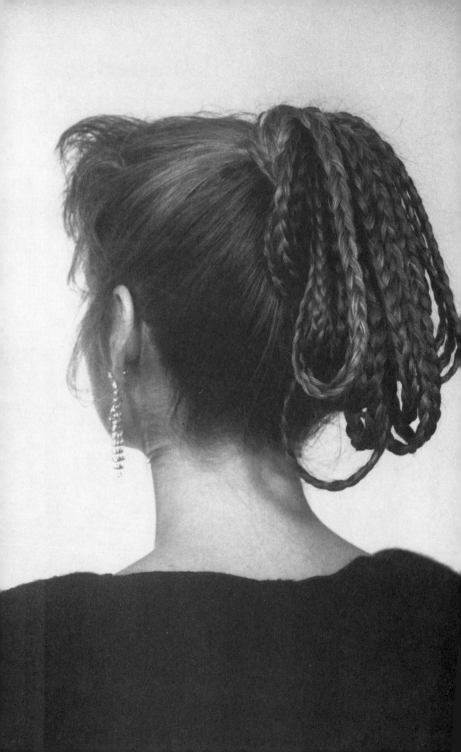

Braided Loops

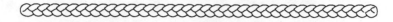

1 Follow directions for Lots of Braids, page 7, steps 1 through 3.

2 Hold all the braids except one and pull upward toward their originating point. Secure each of these braids to the originating point with hairpins.

3 Using the one remaining braid, wrap around the originating point and pinned ends in a circular motion. Tuck the end underneath the wrapped braid and secure with hairpins. •

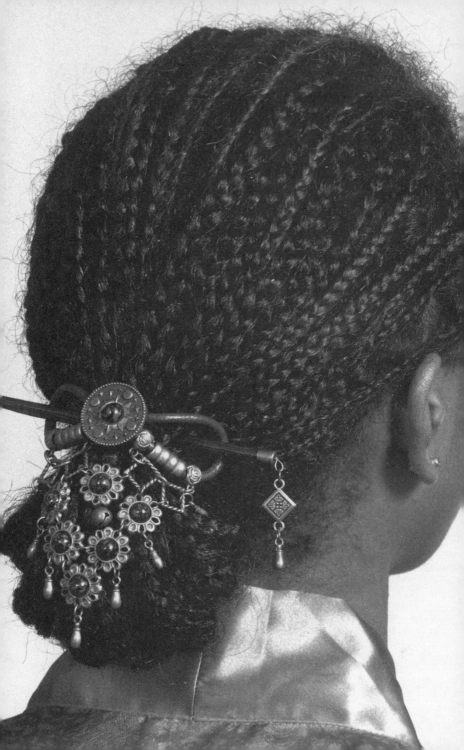

A Bevy of Braids

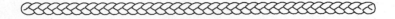

This great look takes time to do, but is well worth the effort.

1   Part a small portion of your hair into a half-inch square.

2   Braid this section, following the Original Braid technique described on page 3.

3   Secure the end with a small band, or tie with string.

4. Repeat steps 1 and 2 until your entire head of hair is braided.

5   Gather hair at the base of your hairline into a ponytail, or you may wish to leave the braids hanging free.

The French

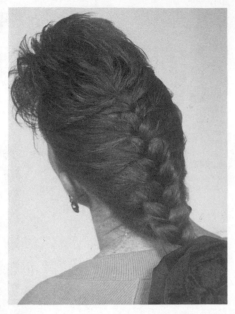

A close-up of the French Braid – crossing the hair over.

A close-up of the French Braid – crossing the hair underneath.

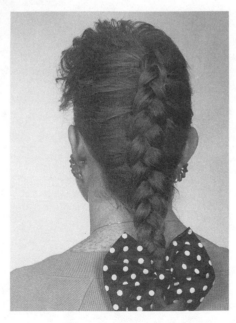

Introduction

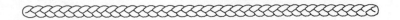

The French Braid is a beautiful braid where you incorporate hair as you progress.

This braiding technique is a skill, and as with most skills, you will improve with practice.

The most difficult part of French braiding is the feeling that you need at least one extra hand. Once you gain control over your fingers and can manipulate the different sections of hair you'll see how easy it can be done.

As you read the directions in this chapter keep in mind that you need to hold the hair in a particular position for each step. With practice, you will learn to hold the hair tighter, which will create a tighter braid.

French braiding can be done either crossing the hair section on top, or underneath as shown in the photos on the left.

You will achieve a smoother and flatter look by crossing the hair on top. In contrast, by crossing the hair underneath, the braid is more visually apparent.

All French Braid hairstyles can be done either way, according to preference.

French Braid • Step-By-Step Instructions

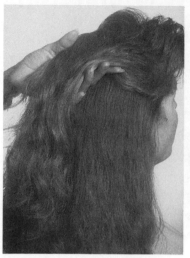

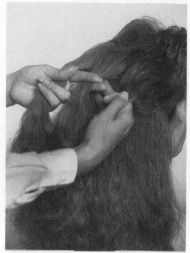

1. Gather a small portion of hair at the center crown of your head.

2. Divide this portion into three equal parts.

3. Proceed to braid your hair using the Original Braid technique as follows:

   • Cross the right over the middle section.

   • Cross the left over the new middle section.

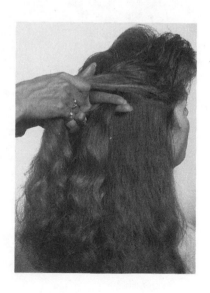

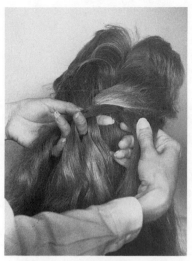

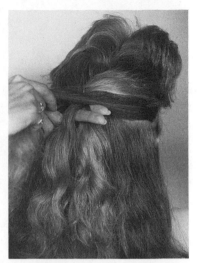

4. Part a thin strip of hair from your right hairline to the braiding area.

5. Add this strip to the right section of hair.

6. Cross the new enlarged right section over the middle section.

7. Part a thin strip of hair from your left hairline to the braiding area.

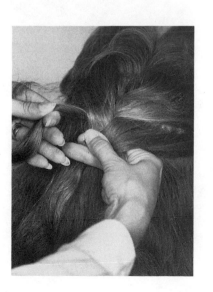

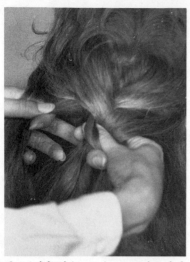

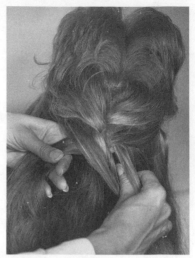

8. Add this strip to the left section of hair.

9. Cross the new enlarged left section over the middle.

10. Repeat steps 4 through 9 until you reach the base of your hairline center back.

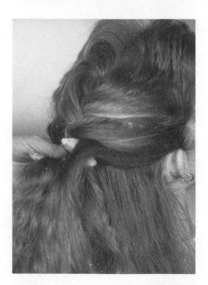

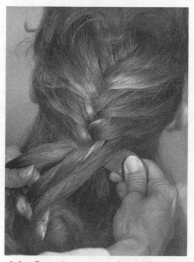
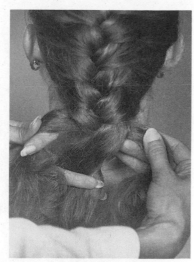

11. Continue to braid using the Original Braid technique described in step 3, until you reach the desired length.

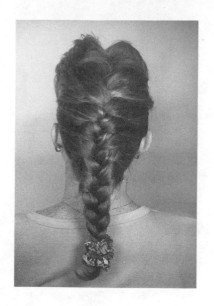

12. Secure with covered elastic band.

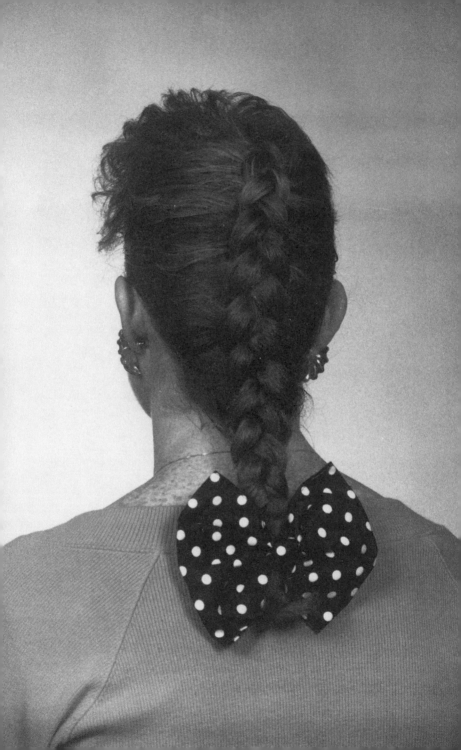

The Single Frenchy I

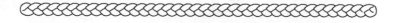

1   Gather a small portion of hair (about the diameter of a pencil) at the crown of your head.

2   Divide this portion into three equal parts.

3   Proceed to braid your hair using the Original Braid technique as follows:

   • Cross the left under the middle section.

   • Cross the right section under the new middle section.

4   Part a thin strip of hair from your left hairline to the braiding area. Add this strip to the left section of hair. Cross the new enlarged left section under the middle section.

   Note: Beginning with step 4 you will be adding hair to the outer left and right sections before you cross to the middle each time.

5   Part a thin strip of hair from your right hairline to the braiding area. Add this strip to the right section of hair. Cross the new enlarged right section under the new middle section.

6   Repeat steps 4 and 5 until you reach the base of your hairline center back.

7   Continue to braid using the Original Braid technique described in step 3, until you reach the desired length.

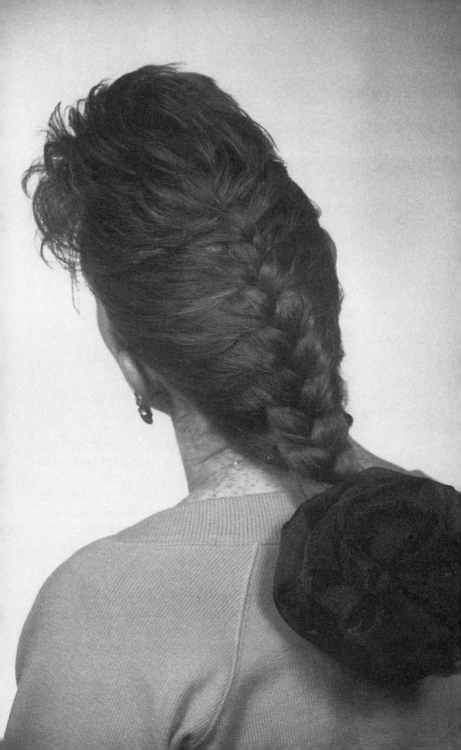

The Single Frenchy II

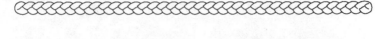

1. Gather a small portion of hair (about the diameter of a pencil) at the crown of your head.

2. Divide this portion into three equal parts.

3. Proceed to braid your hair using the Original Braid technique as follows:

   - Cross the left over the middle section.
   - Cross the right section over the new middle section.

4. Part a thin strip of hair from your left hairline to the braiding area. Add this strip to the left section of hair. Cross the new enlarged left section over the middle section.

   Note: Beginning with step 4 you will be adding hair to the outer left and right sections before you cross to the middle each time.

5. Part a thin strip of hair from your right hairline to the braiding area. Add this strip to the right section of hair. Cross the new enlarged right section over the new middle section.

6. Repeat steps 4 and 5 until you reach the base of your hairline center back.

7. Continue to braid using the Original Braid technique described in step 3, until you reach the desired length.   •

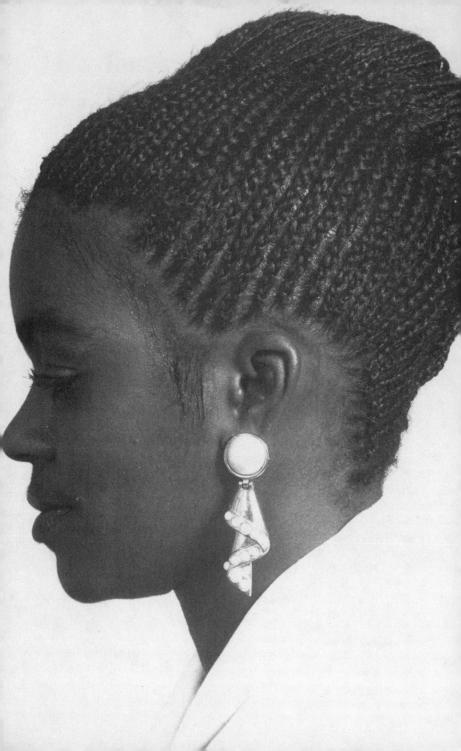

Cornrow

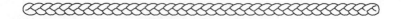

The extensive heritage of this popular braiding style can be directly traced to many tribes throughout the African continent.

You can cornrow your hair in countless directions and patterns to suit the occasion. This hairstyle takes a lot of effort and time, but the result is magnificent.

The directions that follow are for any cornrow hairstyle.

1 Band 4 to 6 sections separately to keep hair free from the working area.

2 Plan the direction that you want the cornrow to lay.

3 Beginning with one section, part your hair in a thin (one-quarter to one-half inch wide) strip in that direction.

4 Proceed to French Braid this strip of hair according to directions for the Single Frenchy I on page 27.

5 Secure the end with a small band or knotted piece of thread. To add beads, wrap a small piece of foil around the end of the braid, thread beads, and crimp the foil to secure them.

6 Repeat steps 2 through 5 until entire head is braided.   •

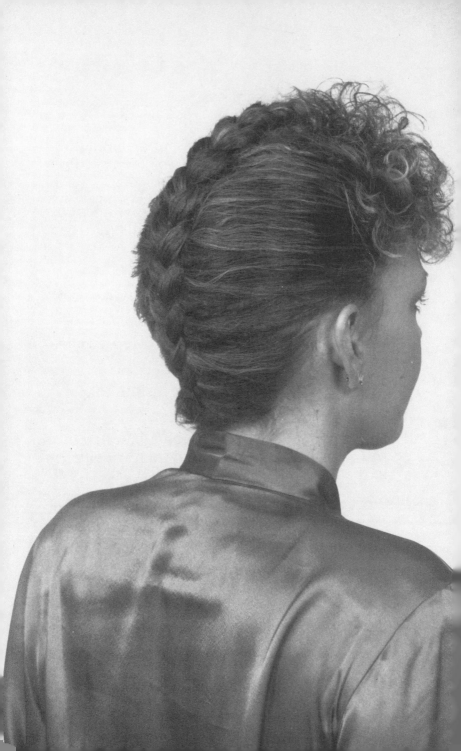

The Upside-Down Frenchy

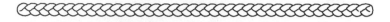

This can be done either crossing under (as shown)or crossing over.

Tip: This braid is easier to do if you lay facedown on the edge of a bed with your head and arms free to move.

1   You will begin braiding the hair at the base of the neck. Gather a small portion of hair (about the diameter of a pencil) at the center base of your head.

2   Divide this portion into three equal parts.

3   Proceed to braid this portion of hair using the Original Braid technique as follows:

   • Cross the left under the middle section.

   • Cross the right section under the new middle section.

4   Part a thin strip of hair from your left hairline to the braiding area.

   • Add this strip to the left section of hair.

   • Cross the new enlarged left section under the middle section.

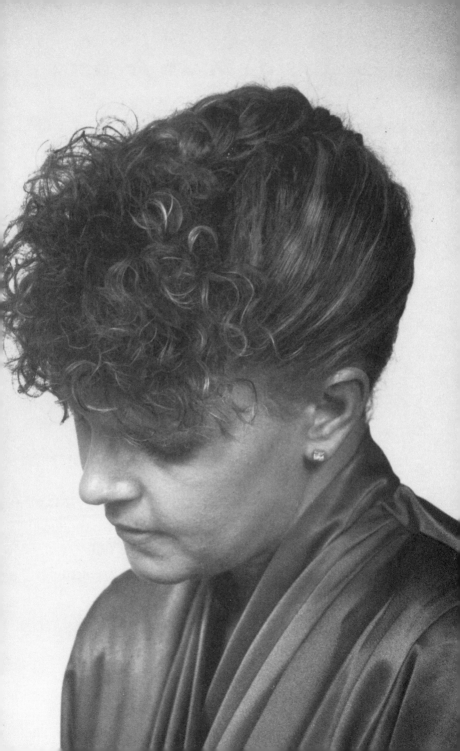

Note: Beginning with step 4 you will be adding hair to the outer left and right sections before you cross to the middle each time.

5   Part a thin strip of hair from your right hairline to the braiding area.

- Add this strip to the right section of hair.
- Cross the new enlarged right section under the new middle section.

6   Repeat steps 4 and 5 until you reach the crown of your head.

7   Continue to braid using the Original Braid technique described in step 3, until you reach the desired length.

8   Tuck the end of braid under itself and use hairpins to secure.   •

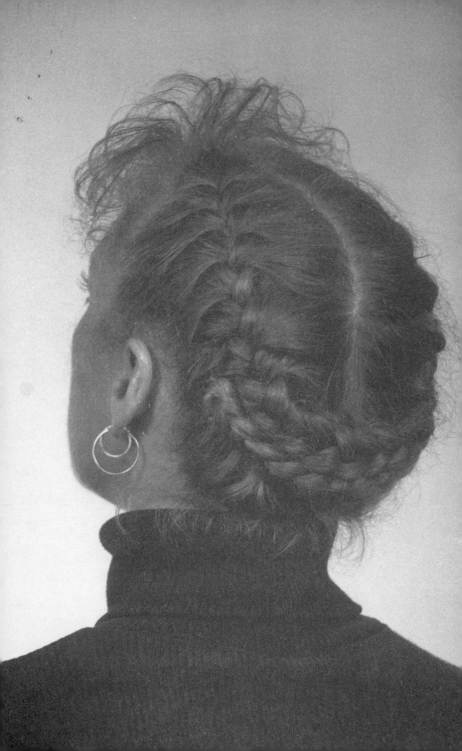

Double-Tucked Frenchy I

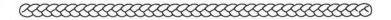

This can be done either crossing over (as shown), or crossing under.

1   Divide your hair into two sections by parting it in the center from the top of your hairline to the base of your hairline.

2   Gather and band the second section (right side of head) while working on section one (left side of head).

3   Gather a small portion of hair at the top side of head.

4   Divide this portion into three equal parts.

5   Proceed to braid this portion of hair using the Original Braid technique as follows:

   • Cross the left over the middle section.

   • Cross the right over the new middle section.

6   Part a thin strip of hair from your left hairline to the braiding area.

   • Add this strip to the left section of hair.

   • Cross the new enlarged left section over the middle section.

7   Part a thin strip of hair from the center part to the braiding area.

- Add this strip to the right section of hair.
- Cross the new enlarged right section over the middle section.

8   Repeat steps 6 and 7 until you reach the base of your hairline or until there is no more hair to add to the braid on the left side.

9   Continue to braid using the Original Braid technique described in step 5, until reaching the entire length. Secure with elastic band.

10 Loosen hair from band on the second section (right side of head).

11 Repeat steps 3, 4, and 5.

12 Part a thin strip of hair from the center part to the braiding area.

- Add this strip to the left section of hair.
- Cross the new enlarged left section over the middle section.

13 Part a thin strip of hair from your right hair-line to the braiding area.

- Add this strip to the right section of hair.
- Cross the new enlarged right section over the middle section.

14 Repeat steps 12 and 13 until you reach the base of your hairline.

15 Continue to braid using the Original Braid technique described in step 5, until reaching the entire length. Secure with elastic band.

16 Pull the end of each braid toward the opposite sides of your head. Lay one braid on top of the other or place the braids horizontally next to each other. Tuck the ends under the braid and secure with hairpins. •

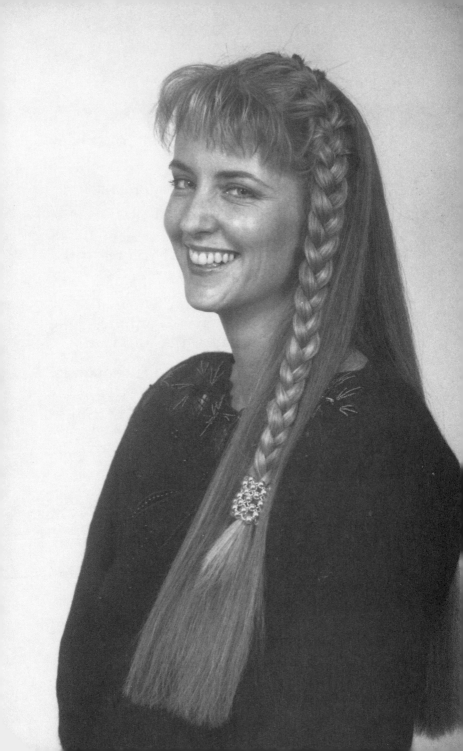

The Headband

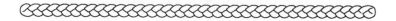

This is the easiest to do on someone else because you can stand on one side and look from above. It then becomes a simple French Braid.

1   Part your hair from ear to ear across the top of your head. Gather the remaining back two-thirds of your hair together and secure with an elastic band.

2   Gather a small portion of hair near the left ear.

3   Divide this small portion into three equal parts.

4   Proceed to braid this portion using the Original Braid technique as follows:

    • Cross the left over the middle section.

    • Cross the right over the new middle section.

5   Gather a thin strip of hair from the part to the braiding area.

    • Add this strip to the left section.

    • Cross the new enlarged left section over the middle section.

6 Gather a thin strip of hair from the temple area hairline to the braiding area.

- Add this strip to the right section.
- Cross the new enlarged right section over the middle section.

7 Repeat steps 5 and 6 until you reach the right ear area.

Each time you repeat these steps, you will be moving upward toward the right ear.

8 Continue to braid the hair using the Original Braid technique described in step 4, until you reach desired length. Secure with band.

9 Take band off the back two-thirds of hair previously held out of the way. •

Frenchy Piggyback

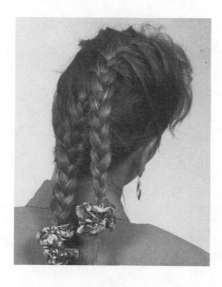

This fun braid is great for the outdoors.

1 Divide your hair into two major sections by parting it horizontally from ear to ear. The top half of the hair from ear to ear and above is section 1. The bottom half of the hair, from ear to ear and below is section 2.

2 Secure section 2 with a band while working with section 1.

3 Braid section 1, using the French Braid technique described on page 22. Braid the entire length of hair, changing to the Original Braid technique when there is no remaining hair to add to the braid. Secure with an elastic band. Clip this braid out of the way.

4 Braid section 2, using the French Braid technique as directed in step 3.

5 Unclip section 1 and let it fall over the top of section 2.

●

43

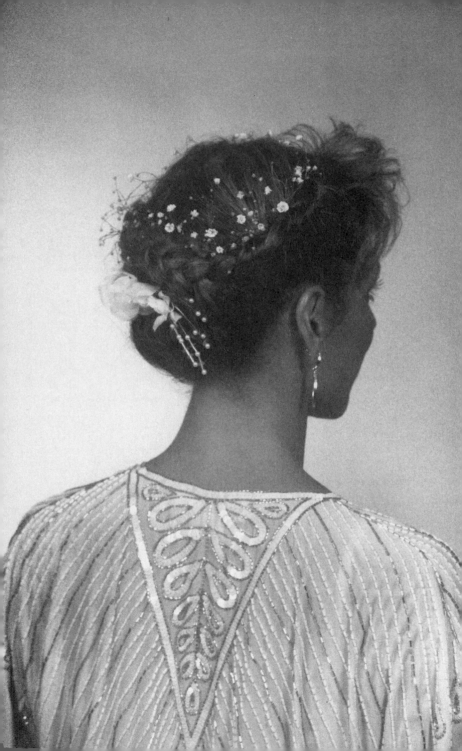

Double Tucked Frenchy II

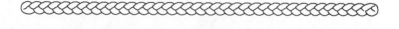

This braid is similar to the Double Tucked Frenchy I on page 37. The major difference is that unlike a true French Braid which gathers and adds hair from each side, the Double-Tucked Frenchy II only gathers hair from one side. Braiding in this fashion creates a braid which makes a "bowl" of your hair, making it ideal to add flowers to the center.

1   Divide your hair into two sections by making a center part from your center forehead to the center back hairline.

2   Secure the right section while working with the left section.

3   Gather a small portion of hair at the top of this section and divide into three working sections.

4   Proceed to braid using the Original Braid technique. Cross the right section over the middle section. Cross the left section over the new middle section.

5   Cross the right section over the new middle section.

6   Part a small strip of hair from your hairline above the temple and add this to the left section.

7 Cross the new enlarged left section over the middle and pull tightly.

8 Keep repeating steps 5, 6, and 7 until you reach the end of your hairline.

Note: Each time you repeat step 6 you will keep adding hair from a lower point of your hairline.

9 Continue to braid, changing to the Original Braid technique until the desired length is reached. Secure with a band. The left section is now braided.

10 Unband the right section and gather a small portion of hair at the top of this section and divide it into three equal working sections.

11 Proceed to braid using the Original Braid technique. Cross the left section over the middle section. Cross the right section over the new middle section.

12 Cross the left section over the new middle section.

13 Part a small strip of hair from your hairline above the temple and add this to the right section.

14 Cross the new enlarged right section over the middle section and pull tightly.

15 Keep repeating steps 12, 13, and 14 until you reach the end of your hairline.

16 Continue to braid using the Original Braid technique until the desired length is reached. Secure with a band.

17 Pull left braid upward, toward the right ear. Tuck the end of braid under itself and secure with hairpins.

18 Pull right braid upward and toward left ear. Tuck end of braid under itself and secure with hairpins.

Optional: At this point you may want to add flowers to your hairstyle. Baby's breath works nicely. •

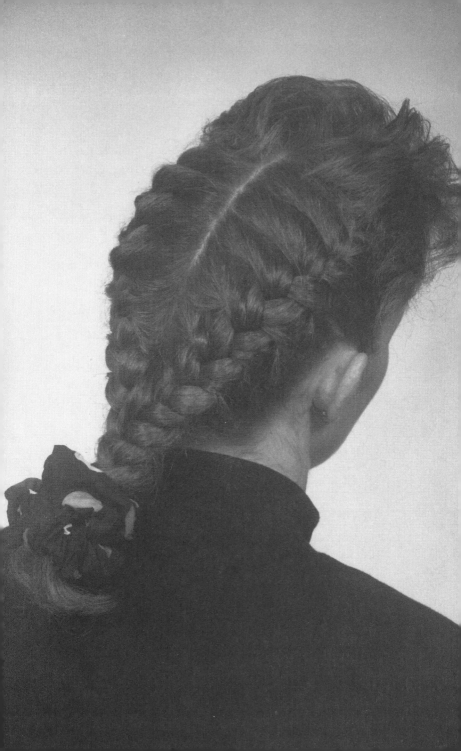

Two-in-One

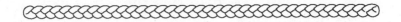

This braid will require an extra set of hands. Find a volunteer!

1   Divide your hair into two equal sections by parting from the top of your head down to the center baseline.

2   Gather and band the right side while working on the left side.

3   Gather a small portion of hair (about the diameter of a pencil) at the top left side of your head.

4   Divide this portion into three equal parts.

5   Proceed to braid your hair using the Original Braid technique as follows:

   • Cross the left over the middle section.

   • Cross the right over the new middle section.

6   Part a thin strip of hair from your left hairline to the braiding area.

   • Add this strip to the left section of hair.

   • Cross the new enlarged left section over the middle section.

7   Part a thin strip of hair from the center part to the braiding area.

- Add this strip to the right section of hair.
- Cross the new enlarged right section over the middle section.

8   Repeat steps 6 and 7 until you reach the base of your hairline.

9   At this point you will need a helping hand. Instruct your helper to hold the three sections you have braided thus far into three separate sections (left, middle, right).

10   The left side is now braided and held firmly in place by your helper.

11   Proceed to braid the right side. First gather a small portion of hair (about the diameter of a pencil) at the top right side of your head.

12   Divide this portion into three equal parts.

13   Proceed to braid your hair using the Original Braid technique as follows:

- Cross the right over the middle section.
- Cross the left over the new middle section.

14   Part a thin strip of hair from your right hairline to the braiding area.

- Add this strip to the right section of hair.
- Cross the new enlarged right section over the middle section.

15 Part a thin strip of hair from the center part to the braiding area.

- Add this to the left section of hair.
- Cross the new enlarged left section over the middle section.

16 Repeat steps 14 and 15 until you reach the base of your hairline.

17 Join the braided right side to the braided left side that is being held. Carefully lay the separate sections (left, middle, right) in your hands on top of the left, middle, and right sections being held by your helper.

- Join the two left sections and hold between your fingers.
- Join the two middle sections and hold.
- Join the two right sections and hold.

Note: You should now have three working sections at the center base of your hairline.

18 Proceed to braid the remaining length of your hair using the Original Braid technique as follows:

- Cross the left over the middle section.
- Cross the right over the new middle section.

19 Secure the end of braid with a covered elastic band.   •

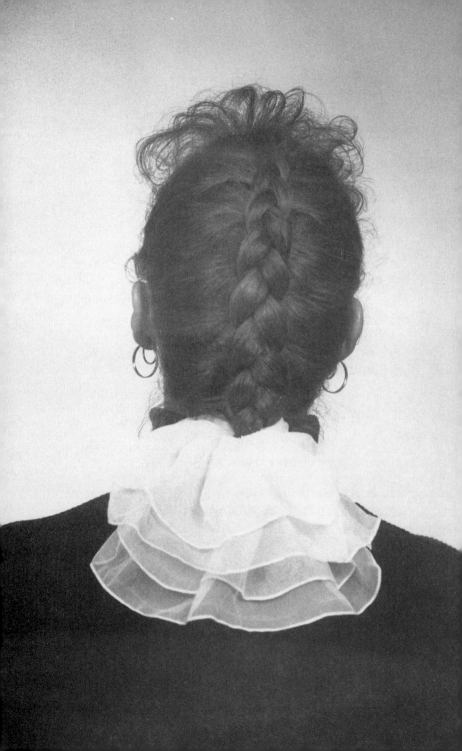

French Ponytail

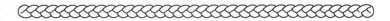

This can be done either crossing under (as shown) or crossing over.

1   Gather a small portion of hair (about the diameter of a pencil) at the center crown of your head.

2   Divide this portion into three equal parts.

3   Proceed to braid your hair using the Original Braid technique as follows:

   • Cross the left under the middle section.

   • Cross the right section under the new middle section.

4   Part a thin strip of hair from your left hairline to the braiding area. Add this strip to the left section of hair. Cross the new enlarged left section under the middle section.

5   Part a thin strip of hair from your right hairline to the braiding area.

   • Add this strip to the right section of hair.

   • Cross the new enlarged right section under the new middle section.

6   Repeat steps 4 and 5 until you reach the base of your hairline center back.

7   Secure the hair with a covered elastic band.   •

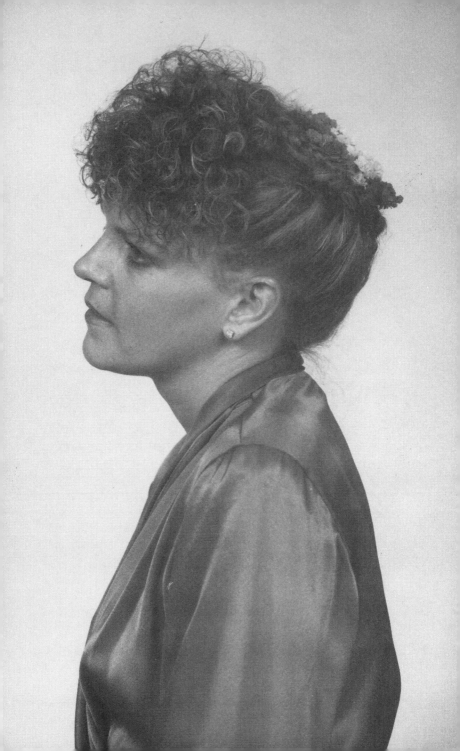

Couronne de Fleurs

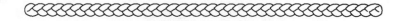

The crown or wreath effect of this braid is achieved by braiding in a circular pattern around the head. The directions are for you to braid someone else's hair. It is a little more difficult to do this braid on yourself but it can be done!

1 Brush hair straight leaving a center part. Position yourself behind and left of the seated person.

2 Gather a small portion of hair (about the diameter of a pencil) at the top left side.

3 Divide this portion into three equal parts.

4 Proceed to braid hair using the Original Braid technique as follows:

   • Cross the left under the middle section.

   • Cross the right section under the new middle section.

5 Part a thin strip of hair from the left hairline to the braiding area.

   • Add this strip to the left section of hair.

   • Cross the new enlarged left section under the middle section.

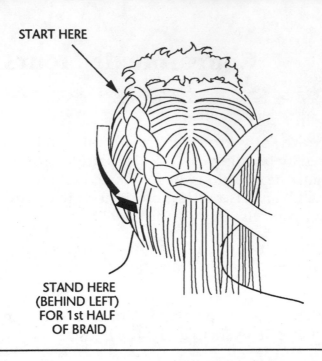

START HERE

STAND HERE
(BEHIND LEFT)
FOR 1st HALF
OF BRAID

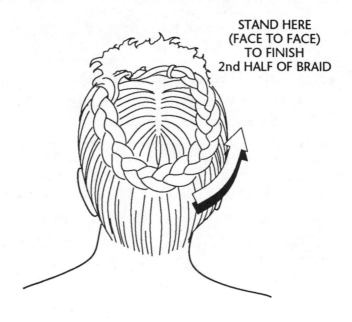

STAND HERE
(FACE TO FACE)
TO FINISH
2nd HALF OF BRAID

6. Part a thin strip of hair from the center part to the braiding area.

   • Add this strip to the right section of hair.

   • Cross the new enlarged right section under the middle section.

7 Repeat steps 5 and 6, moving down the center part with the right sections and further toward the center back hairline with the left sections.

8 When the braid reaches the center back of the head, you will need to move from a behind left position to a left front, face-to-face position. (See diagram at left.)

9 Repeat steps 5 and 6, moving toward the front center part with the right sections and further up the left hairline with the left sections, until you reach the top front of head.

10 Continue to braid remaining length of hair using the Original Braid technique described in step 4. Secure end with a covered elastic band.

11 Curve the loose braid around the front of head to complete a circle. Secure the end with hairpins under the French braided portion.

Small flowers may be added to the inside of the braid with hairpins. •

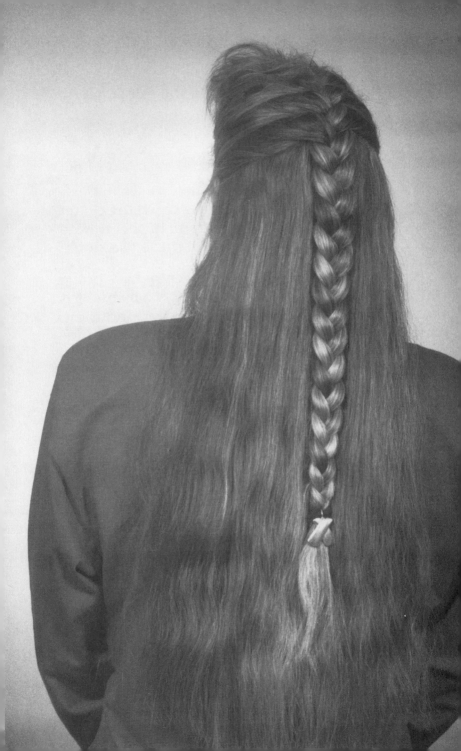

Top Braid & Free

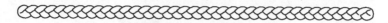

1 Gather a small portion of hair (about the diameter of a pencil) at the top of your head.

2 Divide this portion into three equal parts.

3 Proceed to braid your hair using the Original Braid technique as follows:

   • Cross the left section over the middle section.

   • Cross the right section over the new middle section.

4 Part a thin strip of hair from your left hairline to the braiding area. Add this strip to the left section of hair. Cross the new enlarged left section over the middle section.

5 Part a thin strip of hair from your right hairline to the braiding area.

   • Add this strip to the right section of hair.

   • Cross the new enlarged right section over the middle section.

6 Repeat steps 4 and 5 two more times.

7 Continue to braid this top section of hair using the Original Braid technique described in step 3, until reaching the desired length. Secure with a band.   •

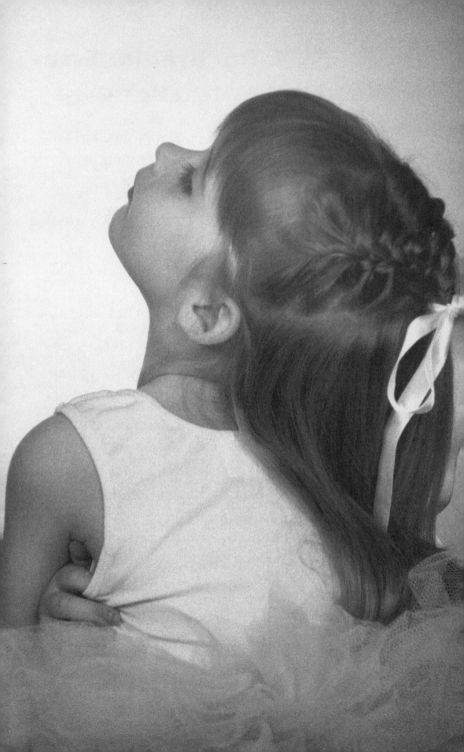

Two Braids & Free

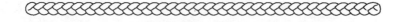

1   Divide your hair into two sections (top and bottom) by parting your hair from ear to ear.

2   Gather and loosely band the long bottom section while working with the top section.

3   Divide the top section into two sections by parting your hair in the center. Gather and loosely band the right section while working with the left section.

4   Starting at the lower left side, gather a small portion of hair and divide into three equal portions.

5   Proceed to braid your hair using the Original Braid technique as follows:

   • Cross the left over the middle section.

   • Cross the right section over the new middle section.

6   Part a thin strip of hair from your left lower partline to the braiding area.

   • Add this strip to the left section of hair.

   • Cross the new enlarged left section over the middle section.

7 Part a thin strip of hair from your right front hairline to the braiding area.

- Add this strip to the right section of hair.
- Cross the new enlarged right section over the middle section.

8 Repeat steps 6 and 7 until you reach the center top of your head. Secure with an elastic band. The left side is now braided.

9 Proceed to French Braid the right side. Unband hair.

10 Starting at the lower right side, gather a small portion of hair and divide it into three equal portions.

11 Proceed to braid your hair using the Original Braid technique as follows.

- Cross the left over the middle section.
- Cross the right section over the new middle section.

12 Part a thin strip of hair from your left front hairline to the braiding area.

- Add this strip to the left section of hair.
- Cross the new enlarged left section over the middle section.

13 Part a thin strip of hair from the right lower partline to the braiding area.

- Add this strip to the right section of hair.
- Cross the new enlarged right section over the middle section.

14 Repeat steps 12 and 13 until reaching the center top of your head. Secure both sections and the previously banded left section together.

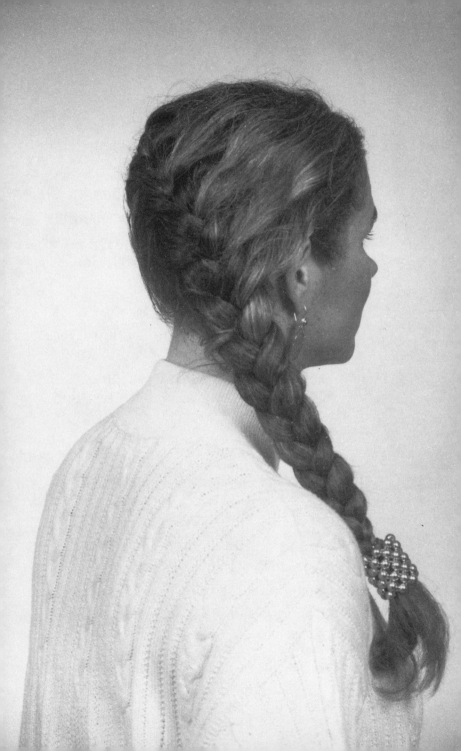

Angle French Braid

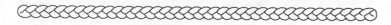

1   Gather a small portion of hair (about the diameter of a pencil) at the top left side of your head.

2   Divide this portion into three equal parts.

3   Proceed to braid your hair using the Original Braid technique as follows:

- Cross the left over the middle section.

- Cross the right section over the new middle section.

4   Part a thin strip of hair from your left hairline to the braiding area. Add this strip to the left section of hair. Cross the new enlarged left section over the middle section.

5   Part a thin strip of hair from your right hairline to the braiding area. Add this strip to the right section of hair. Cross the new enlarged section over the right section.

6   Repeat steps 4 and 5 while you angle from upper left to lower right, until you reach the lower right hairline.

7   Continue to braid the remaining hair using the Original Braid technique described in step 3. Secure with a covered elastic band.   •

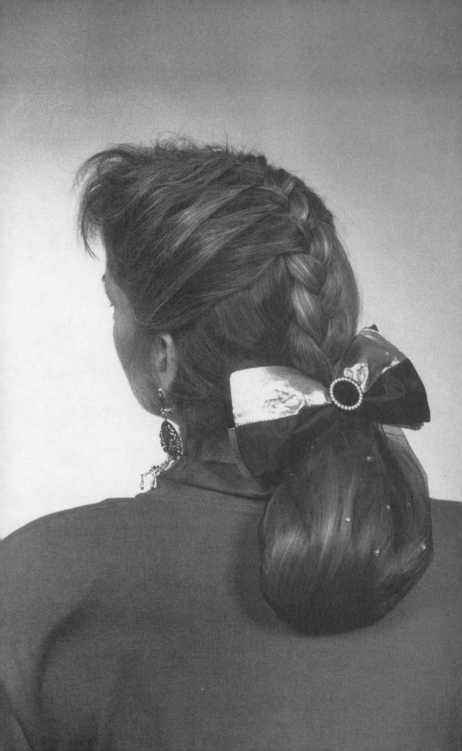

Top Braid into Ponytail

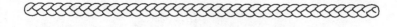

1. Gather a small portion of hair (about the diameter of a pencil) at the top of your head.

2. Divide this portion into three equal parts.

3. Proceed to braid your hair using the Original Braid technique as follows:

   - Cross the left section of the middle section.
   - Cross the right section over the new middle section.

4. Part a thin strip of hair from your left hairline to the braiding area. Add this strip to the left section of hair. Cross the new enlarged left section over the middle section.

5. Part a thin strip of hair from your right hairline to the braiding area. Add this strip to the right section of hair. Cross the new enlarged right section over the middle section.

6. Repeat steps 4 and 5 two more times.

7. Continue to braid this top section of hair using the Original Braid technique described in step 3 until reaching the end of hair.

8. Gather and band the free hanging hair and braided section into a ponytail. Keep the small braided section in the center of your gathered ponytail.   •

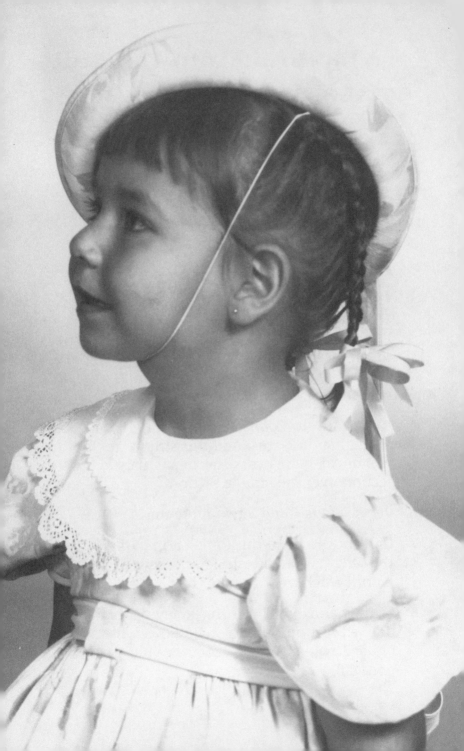

Double Frenchy

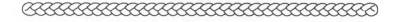

1   Divide hair into two sections by parting it in the center from the top of the hairline to the base of the hairline.

2   Gather and band the right side while working on the left side.

3   Gather a small portion of hair at the top side of head.

4   Divide this portion into three equal parts.

5   Proceed to braid this portion of hair using the Original Braid technique:

  • Cross the left over the middle section.

  • Cross the right over the new middle section.

6   Part a thin strip of hair from your left hairline to the braiding area.

  • Add this strip to the left section of hair.

  • Cross the new enlarged left section over the middle section.

7   Part a thin strip of hair from the center part to the braiding area.

- Add this strip to the right section of hair.
- Cross the new enlarged right section over the middle section.

8   Repeat steps 6 and 7 until you reach the base of your hairline.

9   Continue to braid using the Original Braid technique described in step 5, braiding the entire length of hair. Secure with a band. The left side is now braided.

10 Loosen hair from band on the right side of head.

11 Repeat steps 3, 4, and 5.

12 Part a thin strip of hair from the center part to the braiding area.

- Add this strip to the left section of hair.
- Cross the new enlarged left section over the middle section.

13 Part a thin strip of hair from the right part to the braiding area.

- Add this strip to the right section of hair.
- Cross the new enlarged right section over the middle section.

14 Repeat steps 12 and 13 until reaching the base of your hairline.

15 Continue to braid using the Original Braid technique described in step 5, braiding the entire length of hair. Secure with a band. The right side is now braided. •

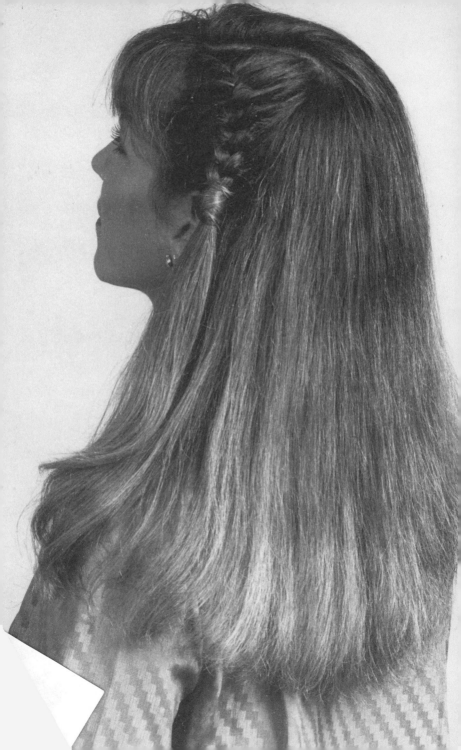

The French Side

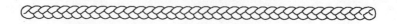

1 Part hair on left side.

2 Gather a very small portion of hair at the upper left corner near the part.

3 Divide this portion into three equal parts.

4 Proceed to braid your hair using the Original Braid technique as follows:

   - Cross the left over the middle section.
   - Cross the right section over the new middle section.

5 Part a very thin strip of hair from your left hairline to the braiding area.

   - Add this strip to the left section of hair.
   - Cross the new enlarged left section over the middle section.

6 Part a very thin strip of hair from your top part line to the braiding area. Add this strip to the right section of hair. Cross the new enlarged right section over the middle section.

7 Repeat steps 5 and 6 three or four more times, moving the braid down toward the left ear.

8 Secure with small band behind left ear. Comb free hanging hair slightly over the braided area.

The Twist

Introduction

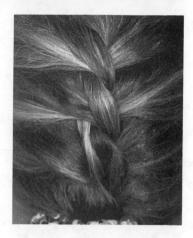

The Twist is named after its appearance. The finished twist looks like twisted rope, even though it is achieved by a crisscrossing technique.

A single twist down the back of your head is a nice look – but be careful – it can *untwist*, depending on the coarseness of your hair.

People who have fine hair or who would like to wear their hair in a single twist (outdoors or to an aerobics class) may want to end the twist in a ponytail at the base of the hairline.   •

The Twist • Step-By-Step Instructions

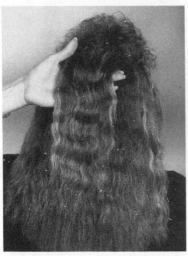

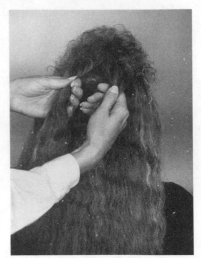

1. Gather a small portion of hair at the center and top of head.

2. Divide that portion into two equal sections.

3. Cross the left section over the right section.

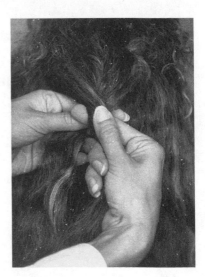

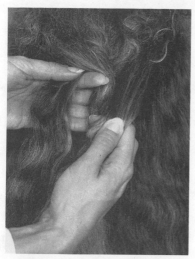

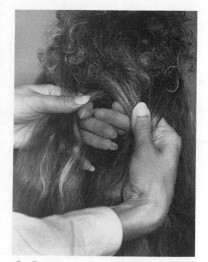

4. Part a new strip of hair (about the diameter of a pencil) from the right hairline to the center crossing area.

• Add this strip to the right section and hold.

5. Part a new strip of hair (about the diameter of a pencil) from the left hairline to the center crossing area.

• Add this strip to the right section and hold.

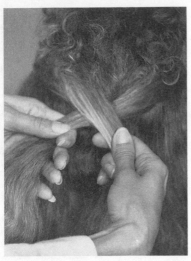

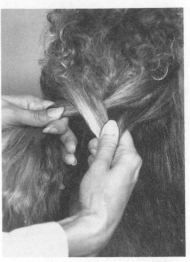

6. Cross the enlarged left section over the enlarged right section.

7. Repeat steps 4 through 6.

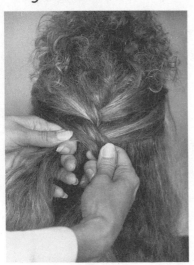

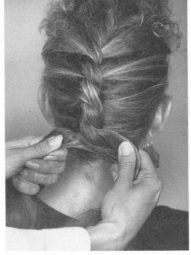

8. Continue until you reach the back center hairline. Secure hair with covered elastic band.

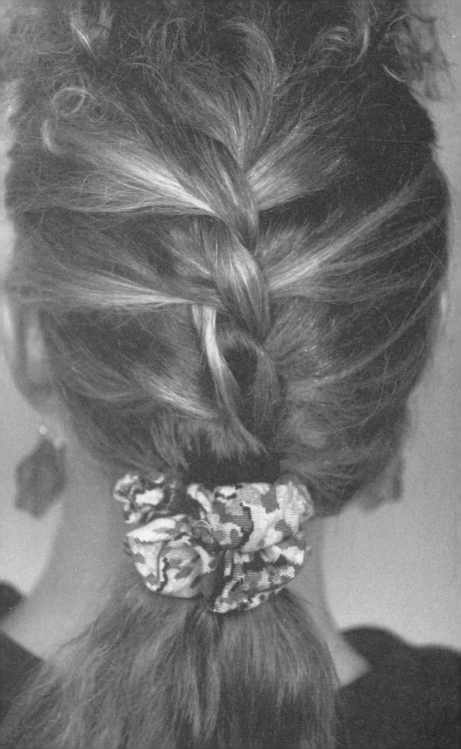

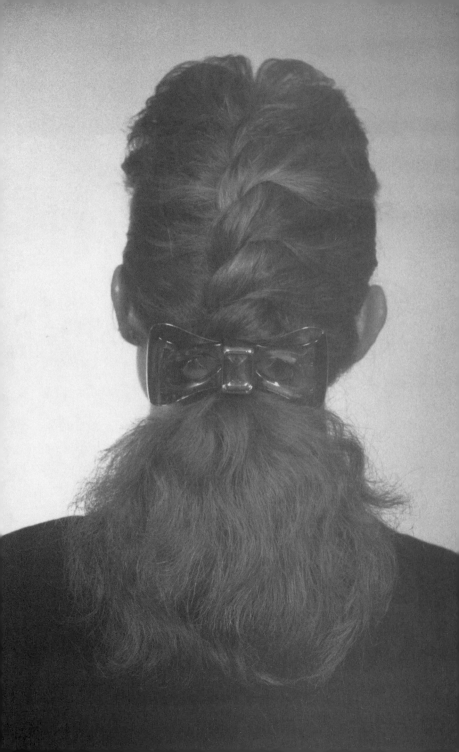

The Single Twist

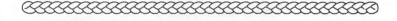

Although this is called a twist because of its appearance, it is actually a crisscrossing technique.

1   Gather a small portion of hair at the center and top of head.

2   Divide that portion into two equal sections.

3   Cross the left section over the right section.

4   Part a new section of hair (about the diameter of a pencil) from the left hairline to the center crossing area.   Add this section to the left section and hold between your fingers.

5   Part a new section of hair (about the diameter of a pencil) from the right hairline to the center crossing area. Add this section to the right section and hold it between your fingers.

6   Cross the enlarged left section over the enlarged right section.

    Note: You will be adding hair to each section before you cross.

7   Proceed to cross the left section over the right section following steps 4 through 6, until you reach the back center hairline of your head.

8   Proceed to cross the left section over the right, following step 3, until you reach the desired length.

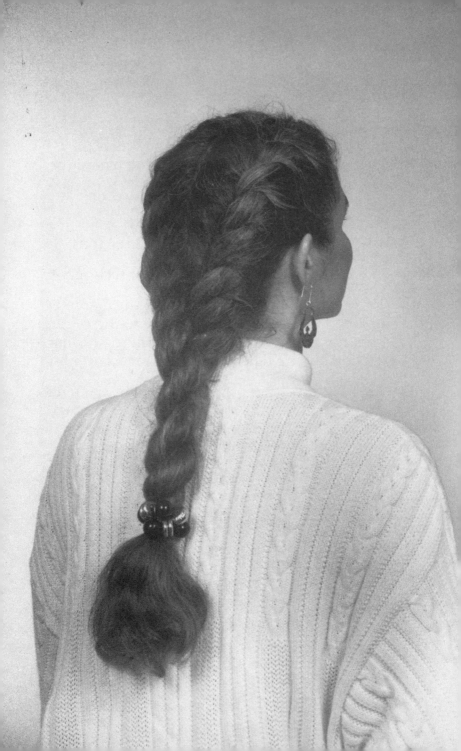

Two-in-One

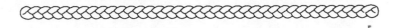

These two twists join together at the base of your head to become one long twist. This hairstyle works best with thick, coarse, long hair. You will need a volunteer to help with this one.

1   Divide your hair into two sections, left and right, by parting the hair down the center from top front to the center back.

2   Loosely band the right side while working with the left side.

3   Gather a small portion of hair at the top left of head.

4   Divide that portion into two equal sections.

5   Cross the left section over the right section.

6   Part a new thin strip of hair (about half an inch wide) from the left hairline to the center crossing area. Add this strip to the left section and hold between your fingers.

7   Part a new thin strip of hair (about half an inch wide) from the center part to the center crossing area. Add this strip to the right section and hold between your fingers.

8   Cross the enlarged left section over the enlarged right section.

Note: You will be adding hair to each section before you cross.

9   Proceed to cross the left sections over the right sections following steps 6 through 8 until you reach the left lower hairline.

10 At this point, your volunteer should hold the twist, keeping the left and right sections separate.

11 Proceed to twist the entire right section. Take the loose band off the right section.

12 Gather a small portion of hair at the top right of your head.

13 Divide that portion into two equal sections.

14 Cross the left section over the right section.

15 Part a new thin strip of hair (about half an inch wide) from the center part to the crossing area.

   • Add this strip to the left section and hold between your fingers.

16 Part a new thin strip of hair (about half an inch wide) from the right hairline to the center crossing area.

- Add this strip to the right section and hold between your fingers.

17 Cross the enlarged left section over the enlarged right section.

18 Proceed to cross the left sections over the right sections following steps 15 through 17, until you reach the right lower hairline.

19 Join the two completed twists together. Place the left and right sections you are holding on top of the left and right sections that your volunteer is holding. Hold the two left sections in one hand and the two right sections in the other hand.

20 Continue crossing the left section over the right section, repeating step 5 until you reach the desired length. Secure with a covered elastic band. •

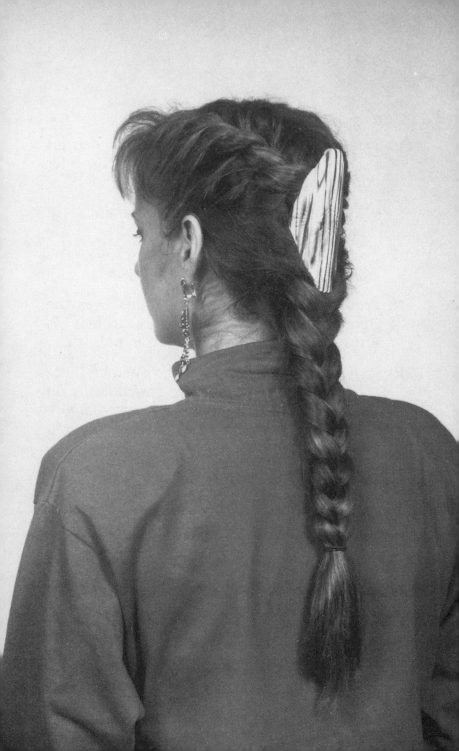

The Original
Two-Sided Twist

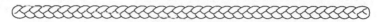

1   Divide hair into two sections, top and bottom,
    by parting your hair from the top left ear to the
    top right ear.

2   Loosely band the bottom section while work-
    ing with the top.

3   Divide the top section of hair into two equal
    portions, left and right, with a center part.
    Loosely band the right section while working
    with the left section.

4   Gather a small portion of hair at the top left
    side of head.

5   Divide that portion into two equal sections.

6   Cross the left section over the right section.

7   Part a new thin strip of hair (about half an inch
    wide) from the left hairline to the center cross-
    ing area.

    • Add this strip to the left section and hold
      between your fingers.

8   Part a new thin strip of hair (about a half an
    inch wide) from the center part to the crossing
    area.

    • Add this strip to the right section and hold
      between your fingers.

9 Cross the enlarged left section over the enlarged right section.

10 Repeat steps 7 through 9 until you reach the center part. Secure with a small covered elastic band. The left twist is now complete.

11 Proceed to twist the top right section. Take the band off the right section.

12 Gather a small portion of hair at the top right side of your head.

13 Divide that portion into two equal sections.

14 Cross the right section over the left section.

15 Part a new thin strip of hair (about half an inch wide) from the right hairline to the center crossing area.

   • Add this strip to the right section and hold between your fingers.

16 Part a new thin strip of hair (about half an inch wide) from the center part to the crossing area.

- Add this strip to the left section and hold between your fingers.

17 Cross the enlarged right section over the enlarged left section.

18 Repeat steps 15 through 17 until you reach the center part.

19 Band the completed right twist with the previously banded left twist.

20 Proceed to braid your hair using the Original Braid technique.

- Divide the free hanging hair into two sections left and right. The sections that have been twisted and banded together will be the middle section.

21 Cross the left over the middle section. Cross the right section over the new middle section.

22 Continue to braid hair repeating step 21 until reaching the desired length. •

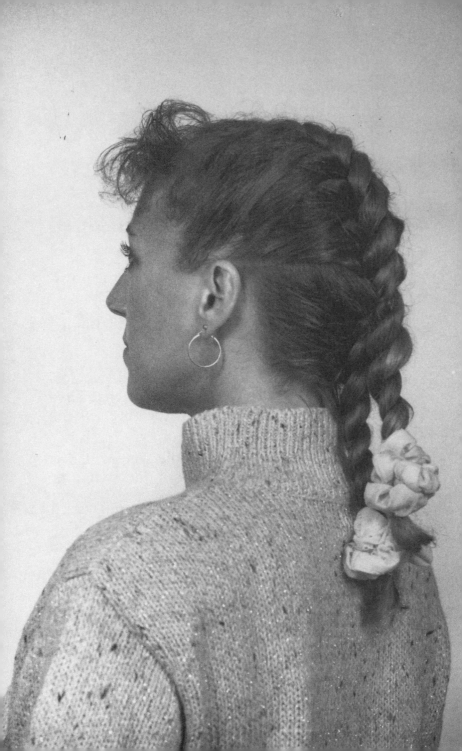

Piggyback Twist

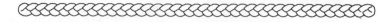

1 Divide your hair into two sections, top and bottom, by parting hair form ear to ear.

2 Loosely band the top section while working on the bottom section.

3 Gather a small portion of hair at the top of the lower section.

4 Divide this portion into two equal sections.

5 Cross the left section over the right section.

6 Part a new thin strip of hair from the left hairline to the center crossing area.

   • Add this section to the left section and hold between your fingers.

7 Part a new thin strip of hair from the right hairline to the center crossing area.

   • Add this section to the right section and hold between your fingers.

8 Cross the enlarged left section over the enlarged right section.

9 Repeat steps 6 through 8 until you reach the back center hairline of your head.

10 Continue crossing the left section over the right section following step 5, until you reach the desired length. Secure end with a covered elastic band. The bottom twist is now completed.

11 Unband the top section.

12 Gather a small portion of hair at the top of your head.

13 Divide this portion into two equal sections.

14 Cross the left section over the right section.

15 Part a new thin strip of hair from the left hairline to the center crossing area.

- Add this section to the left section and hold between your fingers.

16 Part a new thin strip of hair from the right hairline to the center crossing area.

   • Add this section to the right section and hold between your fingers.

17 Cross the enlarged left section over the enlarged right section.

18 Repeat steps 15 through 17 until you reach the back center lower part.

19 Repeat step 5 until you reach the desired length. Secure the end with a covered elastic band. The top twist is now completed.

20 The top twist will lay on top of the bottom twist.   •

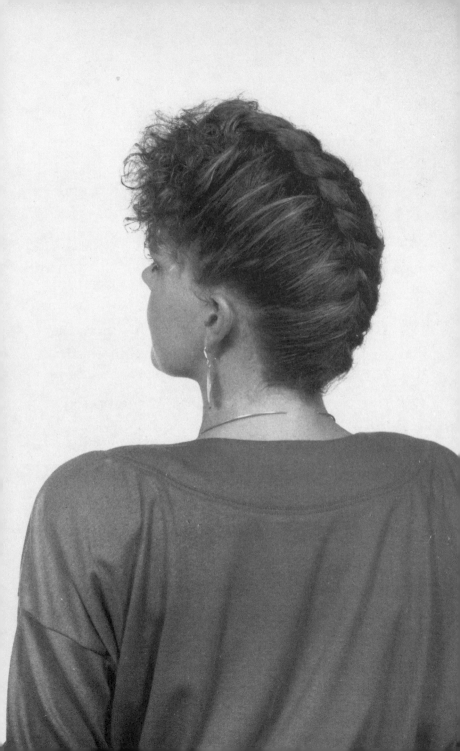

Upside-Down Twist

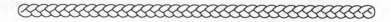

It is easier to do the Upside Down Twist while lying facedown on the edge of a bed or on the floor.

1 Gather a small portion of hair (about the diameter of a pencil) at the base of your hairline.

2 Divide that portion into two equal sections.

3 Cross the left section over the right section.

4 Part a new thin strip of hair from the left hairline to the center crossing area. Add this section to the left section and hold between fingers.

5 Part a new thin strip of hair from the right hairline to the center crossing area. Add this section to the right section and hold between fingers.

6 Cross the enlarged left section over the enlarged right section.

7 Repeat steps 4 through 6 until reaching the top of head.

8 Proceed to cross the left section over the right, repeating step 3, until reaching the length of hair. Secure with a covered elastic band.

9 Tuck the end under itself and secure with hairpins. ●

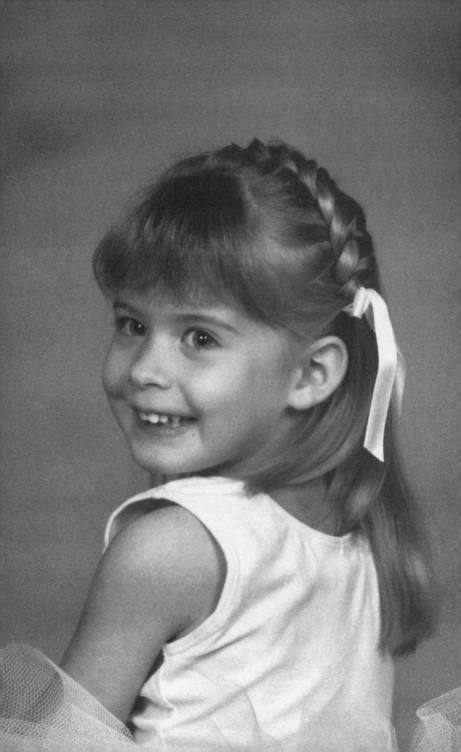

The Twist Headband

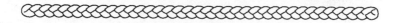

1 Divide your hair into two sections by parting it from ear to ear.

2 Loosely band the bottom section while working on the top section.

3 Gather a small portion of hair (about the diameter of a pencil) near the left ear.

4 Divide this portion into two equal sections.

5 Cross the left section over the right section.

6 Part a new thin strip of hair from the left part-line to the center crossing area. Add this strip to the left section and hold between your fingers.

7 Part a new thin strip of hair from the right hairline to the center crossing area. Add this strip to the right section and hold between your fingers.

8 Cross the enlarged left section over the enlarged right section.

9 Repeat steps 6 through 8 moving upward toward the opposite ear.

10 Secure hair in a covered elastic band near the right ear. Let the ends fall free behind the right ear. •

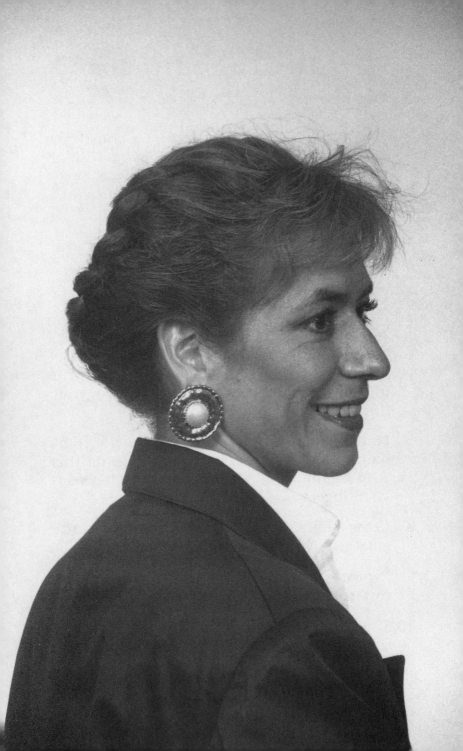

Double Twist & Tucked

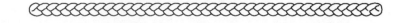

1   Divide hair into two sections, left and right. Part your hair form center top to the base of your hairline.

2   Loosely band the right side while working on the left section.

3   Gather a small portion of hair at the top left side.

4   Divide this portion into two equal sections.

5   Cross the left section over the right section.

6   Part a thin strip of hair from left hairline to center crossing area.

   • Add this strip to the left section and hold it between your fingers.

7   Part a thin strip of hair from center partline to crossing area.

   • Add this strip to the right section and hold it between your fingers.

8   Cross the enlarged left section over the enlarged right section.

9   Repeat steps 6 through 8 until you reach the left lower hairline.

10 Proceed to cross the left section over the right section, repeating step 5 until finishing the entire length of hair. Secure with a band. The left section is now twisted.

11 Unband the right side.

12 Gather a small portion of hair at the top right side.

13 Divide this portion into two equal sections.

14 Cross the right section over the left section.

15 Part a thin strip of hair from the right hairline to center crossing area.

   • Add this strip to the right section and hold between your fingers.

16 Part a thin strip of hair from the center part-line to the crossing area.

   • Add this strip to the left section and hold between your fingers.

17 Cross the enlarged right section over the enlarged left section.

18 Repeat steps 15 through 17 until you reach the right lower hairline.

19 Proceed to cross the right section over the left section, repeating step 5 until reaching the entire length of hair. Secure with a band. The right section is now twisted.

20 Pull the ends of one twist toward the opposite ear. Tuck under and secure with hairpins. Repeat with remaining twist.   •

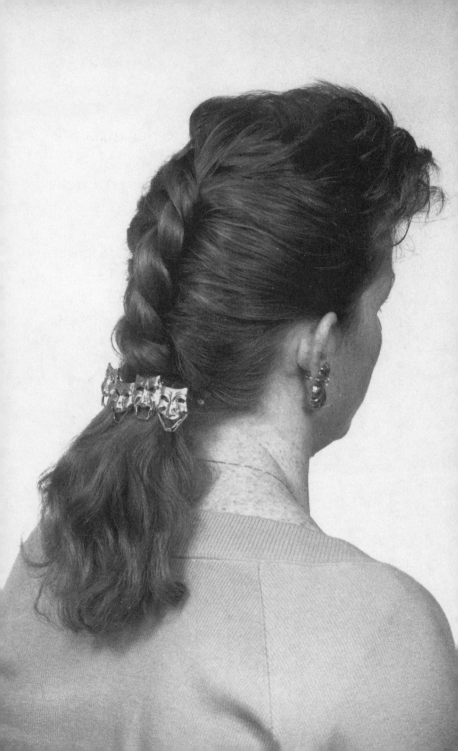

The Twist Ponytail

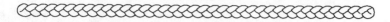

1   Gather a small portion of hair at the center top of your head.

2   Divide this portion into two equal sections.

3   Cross the left section over the right section.

4   Part a new thin strip of hair from the left hairline to the center crossing area.

    • Add this section to the left section and hold between your fingers.

5   Part a new thin strip of hair from right hairline to the center crossing area.

    • Add this section to the right section and hold between your fingers.

6   Cross the enlarged left section over the enlarged right section.

7   Repeat steps 4 through 6 until you reach the back center hairline. Gather at the base of your hairline and secure with covered elastic band.

•

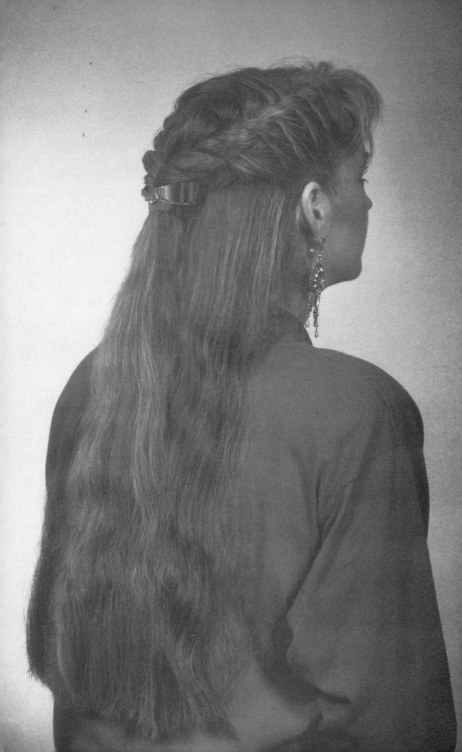

Double Twist & Free

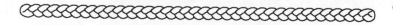

1 Divide your hair into two sections, top and bottom, by parting your hair from the top left ear to the top right ear.

2 Loosely band the bottom section while working with the top.

3 Divide the top section of hair into two equal portions, left and right, with a center part. Loosely band the right section while working with the left.

4 Gather a small portion of hair at the top left side of head.

5 Divide this portion into two equal sections.

6 Cross the left section over the right section.

7 Part a new thin strip of hair (about half an inch wide) from the left partline to the center crossing area.

   • Add this strip to the left section and hold between your fingers.

8 Part a new thin strip of hair (about half an inch wide) from the hairline to the center crossing area.

- Add this strip to the right section and hold between your fingers.

9 Cross the enlarged left section over the enlarged right section.

10 Repeat steps 7 through 9 until you reach the center part. Secure with an elastic band.

11 Proceed to twist the right side. Take the band off the right section.

12 Gather a small portion of hair at the top right side of your head.

13 Divide that portion into two equal sections.

14 Cross the right section over the left section.

15 Part a new thin strip of hair (about a half an inch wide) from the right partline to the center crossing area.

- Add this strip to the right section and hold between your fingers.

16 Part a new thin strip of hair (about a half an inch wide) from the left hairline to the center crossing area.

- Add this strip to the left section and hold between your fingers.

17 Cross the enlarged right section over the enlarged left section.

18 Repeat steps 15 through 17 until you reach the center part.

19 Band the completed right twist with the previously banded left twist. •

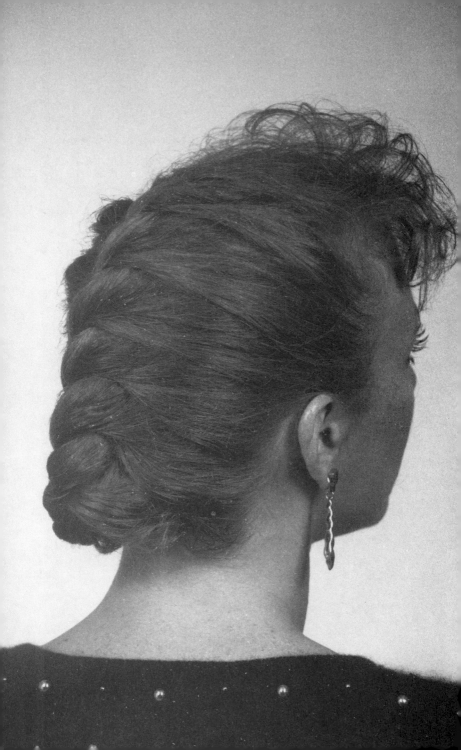

Single Twist & Tucked

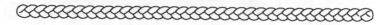

1 Gather a small portion of hair at center top of your head.

2 Divide this portion into two equal sections.

3 Cross the left section over the right section

4 Part a new thin section of hair (about the diameter of a pencil) from the left hairline to the center crossing area. Add this section to the left section and hold between your fingers.

5 Part a new thin section of hair (about the diameter of a pencil) from the right hairline to the center crossing area. Add this section to the right section and hold between your fingers.

6 Cross the enlarged left section over the enlarged right section.

7 Proceed to cross the left section over the right section, following steps 4 through 6, until you reach the back center hairline.

8 Proceed to cross the left section over the right, following step 3, until you reach the length of hair.

9 Tuck the end under itself. Secure with hairpins. ●

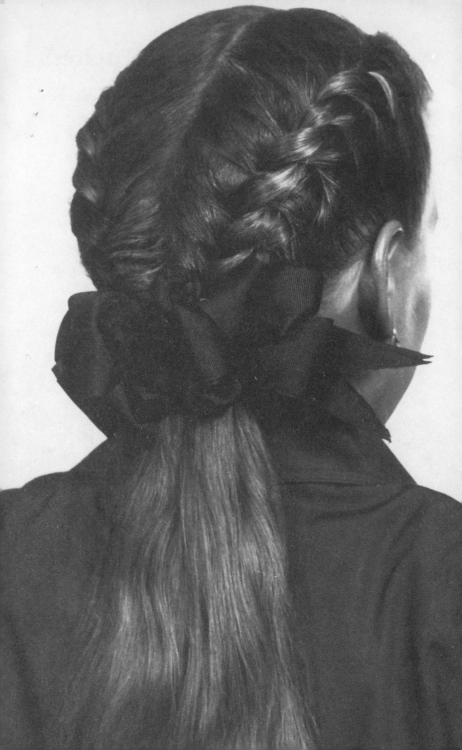

Two-Twist Ponytail

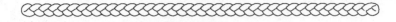

1 Divide your hair into two sections by parting your hair in the center from the top of your head to base of the hairline.

2 Loosely band the right side while working on the left side.

3 Gather a small portion of hair at the top left side.

4 Divide this portion into two equal sections.

5 Cross the left over the right section.

6 Part a thin strip of hair from the left hairline to the center crossing area.

   • Add this strip to the left section and hold between your fingers.

7 Part a thin strip of hair from center partline to crossing area.

   • Add this strip to the right section and hold between your fingers.

8 Cross the enlarged left section over the enlarged right section.

9 Repeat steps 6 through 8 until you reach the left lower hairline.

10 Secure hair with a covered elastic band at the hairline.

11 Unband the right side. Gather a small portion of hair at the top right side.

12 Divide this portion into two equal sections.

13 Cross the right over the left sections.

14 Part a thin strip of hair from the right hairline to center crossing area.

   • Add this strip to the right section and hold between your fingers.

15 Part a thin strip of hair from the center part-line to the crossing area.

   • Add this strip to the left section and hold between your fingers.

16 Cross the enlarged right section over the enlarged left section.

17 Repeat steps 14 through 16 until your reach the right lower hairline.

18 Secure hair with a covered elastic band at hairline.

19 Band or clip the two banded completed twists together.   •

The Fishtail

Introduction

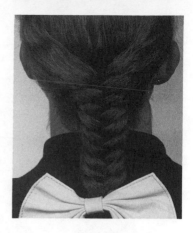

The Fishtail Braid gives your hair the appearance of being intricately woven. This braiding technique is quite simple to master, but rarely seen.

The Fishtail • Step-By-Step Instructions

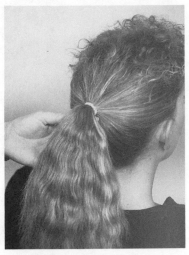

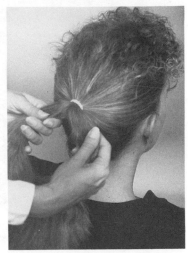

1. *Gather your hair at the center back hairline and band into a ponytail.*

2. *Divide the ponytail into two equal sections with the part being in the center.*

3. *Separate a strand of hair (about the diameter of a pencil) from the outer right side of the right section.*

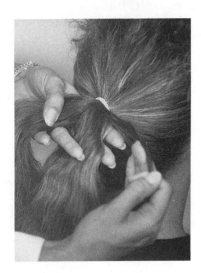

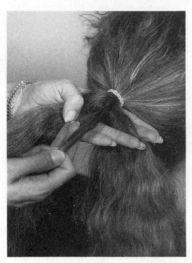

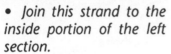

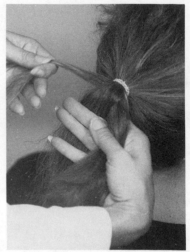

4. Cross this strand over the remaining right section.

   • Join this strand to the inside portion of the left section.

5. Separate a strand of hair (about the diameter of a pencil) from the outer left side of the left section.

   • Cross this strand over the remaining left section.

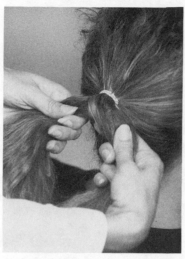

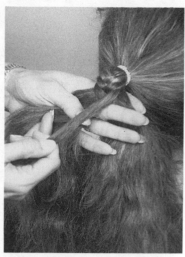

6. Join this strand to the inside portion of the right section.

7. Repeat steps 3 through 6 until reaching the desired length.

8. Secure the end with a covered elastic band.

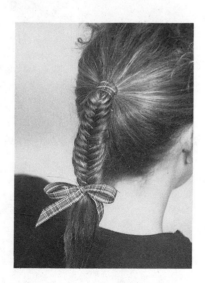

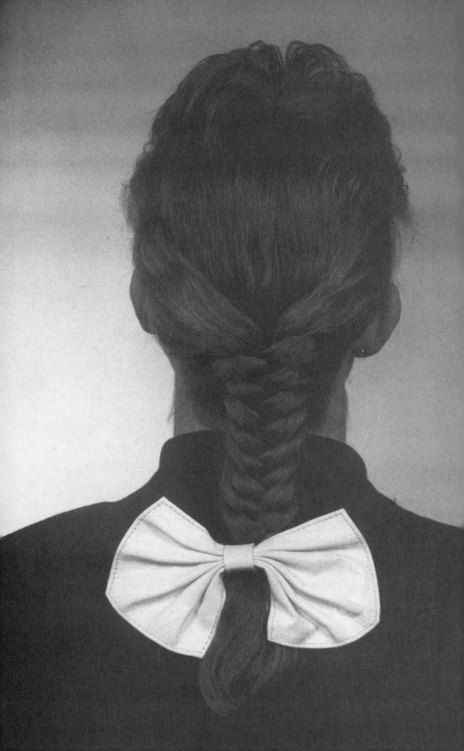

The Fishtail

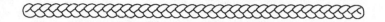

Unlike the French Braid, the Fishtail has two, not three, working sections.

1 Gather your hair at the center back hairline and divide it into two equal sections with the part being in the center.

2 Separate a strand of hair (about the diameter of a pencil) from the outer right side of the right section.

   - Cross this strand over the remaining right section.

   - Join this strand to the inside portion of the left section.

3 Separate a strand of hair (about the diameter of a pencil) from the outer left side of the left section.

   - Cross this strand over the remaining left section.

   - Join this section to the inside portion of the right section.

4 Repeat steps 2 and 3 until reaching the desired length.

5 Secure the end with a covered elastic band. •

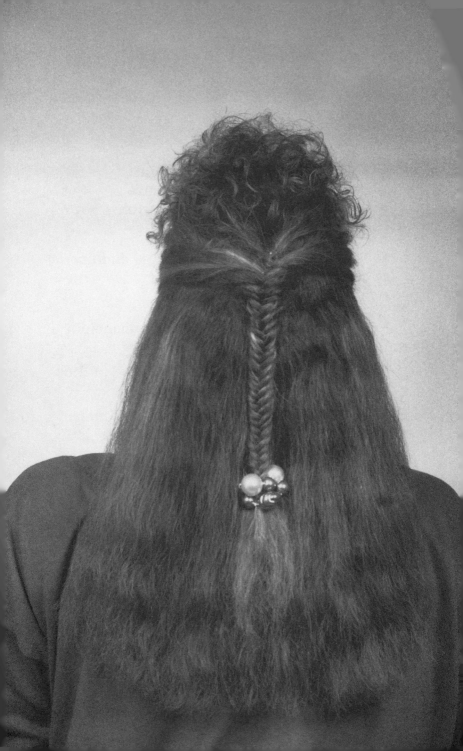

Fishtail in Long Hair

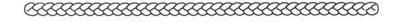

1   Divide your hair into two sections, top and bottom, by parting the hair from top left ear to top right ear.

2   Loosely band the lower section while working with top section.

3   Gather the hair at top of your head and divide it into two equal sections, with the part in the center.

4   Separate a strand of hair (about the diameter of a pencil) from the outer right side of the right section. Cross this strand over the remaining right section. Join this strand to the inside portion of the left section.

5   Separate a strand of hair (about the diameter of a pencil) from the outer left side of the left section. Cross this strand over the remaining left section. Join this strand to the inside portion of the right section.

6   Repeat steps 4 and 5 until finishing the length of hair. Secure with covered elastic band.

7   Take band off the lower section and allow hair to hang freely with the braid in the center.   •

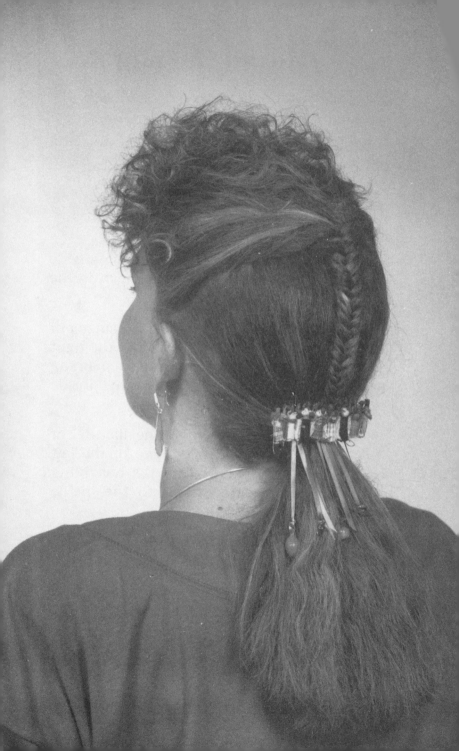

The Fishtail into a Ponytail

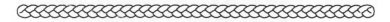

1 Divide your hair into two sections, top and bottom, by parting the hair from the top left ear to the top right ear.

2 Loosely band the lower section while working with the top section.

3 Gather your hair at top of head and divide into two equal sections, with the part being in the center.

4 Separate a strand of hair (about the diameter of a pencil) from the outer right side of the right section. Cross this strand over the remaining right section. Join this strand to the inside portion of the left section.

5 Separate a strand of hair (about the diameter of a pencil) from the outer left side of the left section. Cross this strand over the remaining left section. Join this strand to the inside portion of the right section.

6 Repeat steps 4 and 5 until finishing the length of hair. Secure with a covered elastic band.

7 Gather all hair at lower center hairline and band together, keeping the braided portion in the center. •

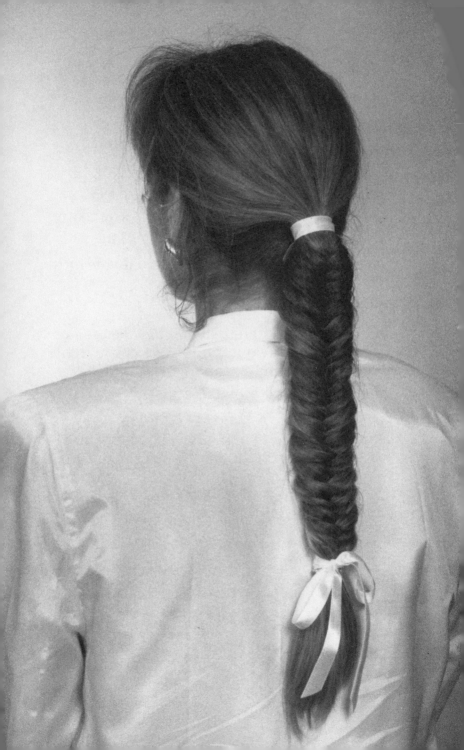

The Pony Fishtail

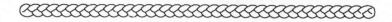

1   Gather your hair at center back hairline into a ponytail. Secure with a covered elastic band.

2   Divide the ponytail into two equal sections.

3   Separate a strand of hair (about the diameter of a pencil) from the outer right side of the right section.

- Cross this strand over the remaining right section.

- Join this strand to the inside portion of the left section.

4   Separate a strand of hair (about the diameter of a pencil) from the outer left side of the left section.

- Cross this strand over the remaining left section

- Join this strand to the inside portion of the right section.

5   Repeat steps 3 and 4 until reaching the desired length.

6   Secure the end with a covered elastic band.   •

The Roll

Introduction

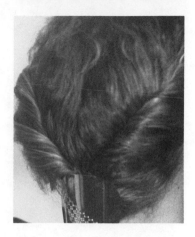

The rolling method of hairstyling is described in detail on the following pages.

The Roll creates a beautiful sleek look that can go from the office to a party with ease.

You may find it easier to do this rolling technique on wet hair as it tends to stay rolled tighter.

The Roll • Step-By-Step Instructions

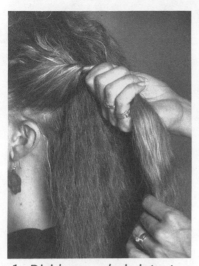

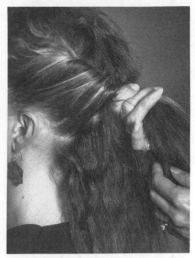

1. Divide your hair into two equal sections by parting from the top center of your head to center lower hairline. Loosely band the right side while working with the left side.

2. Gather a small portion of hair at the upper left side.

3. Roll or twist hair in a clockwise motion, approximately three full turns. Hold.

4. Part a new section of hair from left hairline to rolling area.

   • Add this section to twisted/rolled section being held.

5. Roll or twist enlarged section of hair in a clockwise motion, approximately three full turns. Hold.

6. Repeat steps 4 and 5 until you reach the center back hairline.

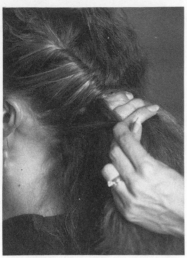

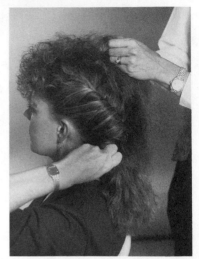

7. *Secure in place with large a clip, or have a volunteer hold in place for later use .*

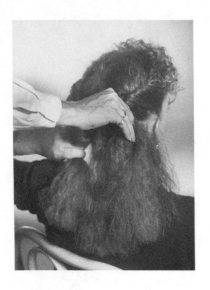

8. *Proceed to roll the right side. Gather a small portion of hair at the upper right side.*

9. *Roll or twist the hair in a counterclockwise motion, approximately three full turns. Hold.*

10. *Part a new section of hair from the right hairline to the rolling area.*

   • *Add this section to the rolled section in your hands.*

11. *Roll or twist enlarged section of hair in a counterclockwise motion, appproximately three full turns. Hold.*

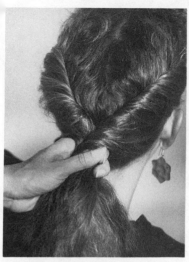

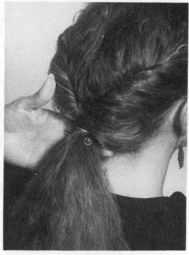

12. Repeat steps 10 and 11 until you reach the center back hairline.

13. Band the rolled right side to the previously rolled left side being held or clipped.

14. Use a decorative hair clip to cover the elastic band.

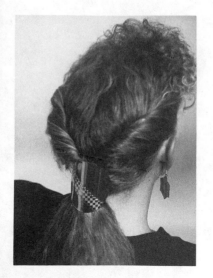

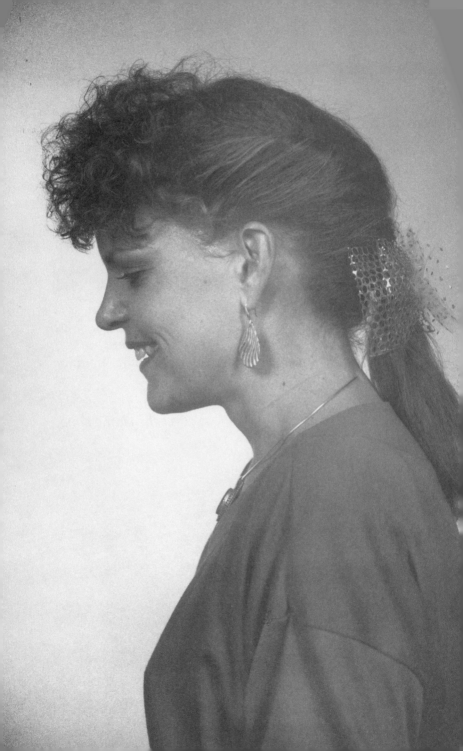

Side Rolls

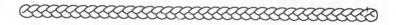

1   Divide your hair into two equal sections by parting from the top center of your head to the center lower hairline.

2   Loosely band the right side while working with the left side.

3   Gather a small portion of hair at the upper left side.

4   Roll or twist the hair in a clockwise motion, approximately three full turns. Hold.

5   Part a new section of hair from left hairline to rolling area.

   • Add this section to the twisted section being held.

6   Roll or twist enlarged section of hair in a clockwise motion, approximately three full turns. Hold.

7   Repeat steps 5 and 6 until you reach the center back hairline. Secure in place with a large clip (or have volunteer hold in place) until later.

8   Proceed to roll the right side. Gather a small portion of hair at the upper right side.

9 Roll or twist the hair in a counterclockwise motion, approximately three full turns. Hold.

10 Part a new section of hair from right hairline to rolling area.

   • Add this section to twisted section being held.

11 Roll or twist enlarged section of hair in a counterclockwise motion, approximately three full turns. Hold.

12 Repeat steps 10 and 11 until you reach the center back hairline.

13 Band the rolled right side to the previously rolled left side being held or clipped with a covered elastic band.   •

The Single Roll

1 Gather a small portion of hair (about two inches wide) at the very top center of your head.

2 Proceed to roll or twist the hair in a clockwise motion, approximately three full turns.

3 Part a thin strip of hair from the right hairline to the center rolling area.

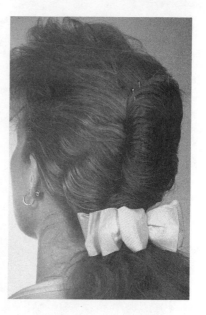

4 Part a thin strip of hair from the left hairline to the center rolling area.

5 Add these two strips to the previously rolled or twisted hair.

6 Roll or twist the enlarged portion in a clockwise motion, approximately three full turns.

7 Repeat steps 3 through 6 until you reach the base of the hairline center back.

8 Band the hair together at the hairline with a covered elastic band.   •

Braid
Free

Introduction

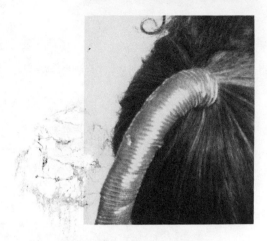

The hairstyles in this chapter are ones where you do not braid, twist, or roll your hair.

These styles are easy, quick, and fun to do to your hair.

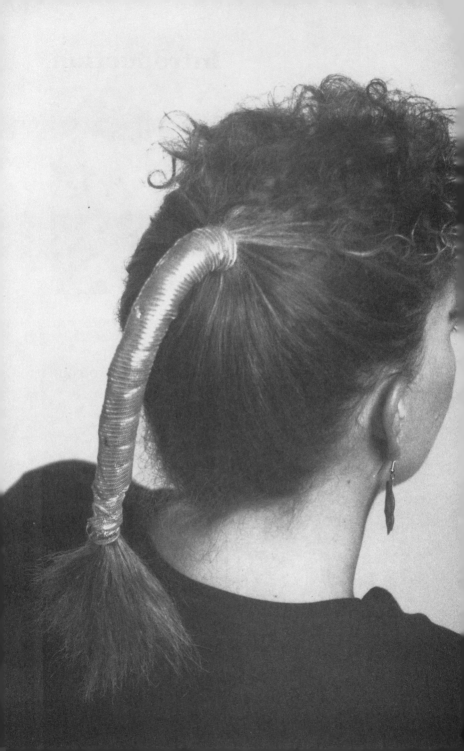

The Slicker

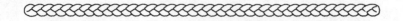

1 Gather all your hair in a high ponytail near the crown of your head. Secure with a band.

2 Gather the bottom of the free hanging ponytail and secure with a band.

3 Tie the end of a long wide ribbon to the base of the ponytail.

4 Proceed to wind the ribbon down the entire length of the ponytail until you reach the banded end.

5 Cut the end of the ribbon down the center about three inches long. Split the ends of the ribbon and tie in a knot around the ponytail. Tuck loose ends under.   •

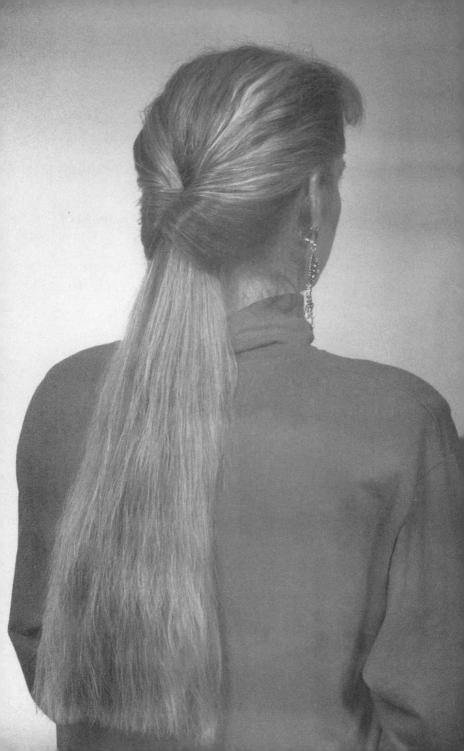

The Tuck-Through

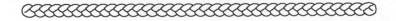

1 Gather your hair in a ponytail at the base of the neck. Secure with a covered elastic band.

2 Make a center part in the hair slightly above covered band.

3 Gather the free hanging ponytail and lift upward.

4 Push the ponytail through the center part.

5 Pull the ponytail through the divided hair tightly from underneath.   •

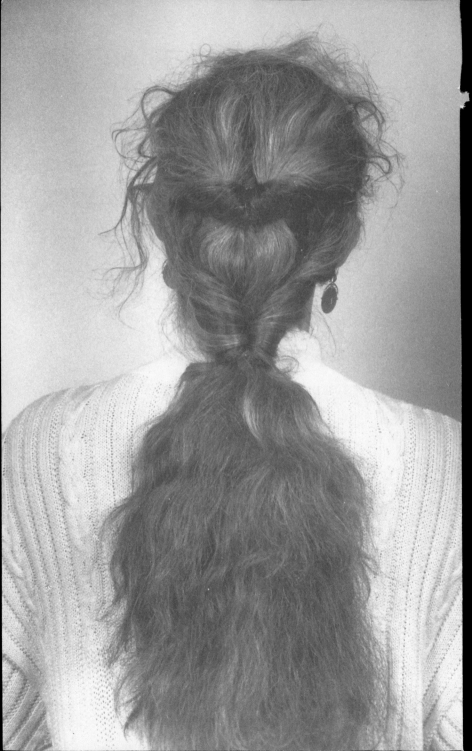

The Multi-Tuck-Through

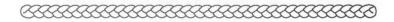

This can be done with two tucks or more, depending on the thickness and length of your hair.

1 Gather the top portion of your hair in a ponytail at the crown of your head. Secure with a covered elastic band.

2 Make a center part in hair slightly above the covered band.

3 Gather the free hanging ponytail and lift upward.

4 Push the ponytail through the center part.

5 Pull the ponytail through the divided hair tightly from underneath.

6 Gather the hair in a ponytail at the base of your neck. Secure with a covered elastic band.

7 Repeat steps 2 through 5.   •

Unbraid

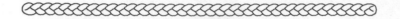

Brushing Out

Remove the covered elastic bands and gently loosen the braid(s) with your fingers.

Gently brush hair to remove large tangles before washing and restyling hair.

To Crimp Your Hair

Braid your hair in any of the braided styles while your hair is wet.

Unband the hair when it is completely dry. Loosen the braid with your fingers and gently brush out. Your hair will be nicely crimped.

Caution

To avoid unecessary breakage of your hair, do not leave your hair braided in a tight style more than a day at a time.